Fifty Neurological Cases from the National Hospital

FIFTY NEUROLOGICAL CASES FROM THE NATIONAL HOSPITAL

Edited by

Adrian Wills BSc (Hons) MB BS MD MRCP
Locum Consultant Neurologist
Department of Neurology
King's College Hospital
London

C David Marsden DSc FRCP FRS
Dean and Professor of Neurology
Institute of Neurology
National Hospital for Neurology and Neurosurgery
Queen Square
London

informa

healthcare

New York   London

Informa Healthcare USA, Inc.
52 Vanderbilt Avenue
New York, NY 10017

10 9 8 7 6 5 4 3 2

International Standard Book Number-10: 1-8531-7677-X (Softcover)
International Standard Book Number-13: 978-1-8531-7677-7 (Softcover)

Visit the Informa Web site at
www.informa.com

and the Informa Healthcare Web site at
www.informahealthcare.com

CONTENTS

LIST OF CONTRIBUTORS

Kailash Bhatia MB BS MD DM, Senior Lecturer and Consultant Neurologist, National Hospital for Neurology and Neurosurgery, Queen Square, London WC1N 3BG

Peter Brown MB BChir MD MRCP, Consultant Neurologist, National Hospital for Neurology and Neurosurgery, Queen Square, London WC1N 3BG; and Middlesex Hospital and University College Hospital, London W1N 8AA

H Alan Crockard MB BCh BAO FRCS FRCS Ed, Consultant Neurosurgeon, National Hospital for Neurology and Neurosurgery, Queen Square, London WC1N 3BG

Charles A Davie MB ChB MRCP MD, Lecturer, National Hospital for Neurology and Neurosurgery, Queen Square, London WC1N 3BG

Christopher J Earl MB BS MD FRCP, Honorary Consultant Physician in Neurology, Moorfields Eye Hospital, Middlesex Hospital and National Hospital for Neurology and Neurosurgery, Queen Square, London WC1N 3BG

Nicholas C Fox MRC Clinician Scientist, Dementia Research Group, National Hospital for Neurology and Neurosurgery, Queen Square, London WC1N 3BG

Richard S J Frackowiak MA MD DSc FRCP, Dean, Institute of Neurology, Professor and Head, Wellcome Department of Cognitive Neurology, Institute of Neurology, Queen Square; Consultant Neurologist, National Hospital for Neurology and Neurosurgery, Queen Square, London WC1N 3BG

Peter J Goadsby MB BS PhD DSc MD FRACP FRCP, Wellcome Research Fellow and Professor of Neurology, National Hospital for Neurology and Neurosurgery, Queen Square, London WC1N 3BG

Michael G Hanna BSc (Hons) MB ChB (Hons) MRCP MD, Consultant Neurologist and Senior Clinical Lecturer, National Hospital for Neurology and Neurosurgery, Queen Square, London WC1N 3BG

Michael J G Harrison MA BM BCh DM FRCP, Professor in Clinical Neurology, University College and London School of Medicine; Consultant Neurologist, National Hospital for Neurology and Neurosurgery, Queen Square, London WC1N 3BG

John M Land BSc PhD BM BCh MBA, Consultant Chemical Pathologist, National Hospital for Neurology and Neurosurgery, Queen Square, London WC1N 3BG

Andrew J Lees MB BS MD FRCP, Consultant Neurologist, National Hospital for Neurology and Neurosurgery, Queen Square, London WC1N 3BG; and Middlesex Hospital and University College Hospital, London W1N 8AA

Nicholas A Losseff MB BS MRCP, Neurology Specialist Registrar, King's College Hospital, London SE5 9RS

Hadi Manji MB BChir MA MD FRCP, Consultant Neurologist, National Hospital for Neurology and Neurosurgery, Queen Square, London WC1N 3BG

C David Marsden DSc FRCP FRS, Dean and Professor of Neurology, Institute of Neurology, National Hospital for Neurology and Neurosurgery, Queen Square, London WC1N 3BG

W Ian McDonald MB ChB PhD FRCP FRCOphth FRACP, Professor and Head, University Department of Clinical Neurology, Institute of Neurology; Honorary Consultant Physician, National Hospital for Neurology and Neurosurgery, Queen Square, London WC1N 3BG, and Moorfields Eye Hospital, London EC1V 2PD

David H Miller MD FRACP FRCP, Professor of Clinical Neurology, Department of Clinical Neurology, Institute of Neurology, National Hospital for Neurology and Neurosurgery, Queen Square, London WC1N 3BG

John A Morgan-Hughes BA MB BChir MD FRCP, Consultant Physician Emeritus; and Honorary Research Fellow, Institute of Neurology and National Hospital for Neurology and Neurosurgery, Queen Square, London WC1N 3BG

Gordon Plant MB BChir MA MD FRCP, Consultant Neurologist, National Hospital for Neurology and Neurosurgery, Queen Square, London WC1N 3BG

Mary M Reilly MB BCh BAO MD MRCPI, Senior Registrar in Neurology, Department of Neurology, Guy's Hospital, London SE1 9RT

Martin N Rossor MB BChir MA MD FRCP, Consultant Neurologist, National Hospital for Neurology and Neurosurgery, Queen Square, London WC1N 3BG

Peter Rudge MB BS FRCP, Consultant Neurologist, MRC Neuro-otology Unit, National Hospital for Neurology and Neurosurgery, Queen Square, London WC1N 3BG; Northwick Park Hospital, Harrow HA1 3UJ

John W Scadding MB BS MD FRCP, Consultant Neurologist, National Hospital for Neurology and Neurosurgery, Queen Square, London WC1N 3BG

Francesco Scaravilli MD PhD FRCPath, Professor of Neuropathology and Honorary Consultant Neuropathologist, Institute of Neurology, National Hospital for Neurology and Neurosurgery, Queen Square, London WC1N 3BG

Raad A W Shakir MB ChB MSc FRCP, Consultant Neurologist, Regional Neurosciences Centre, Charing Cross Hospital, London W6 8RF; Central Middlesex Hospital, London NW10 7NS

Simon D Shorvon MB BChir MD FRCP, Professor of Clinical Neurology, Institute of Neurology, National Hospital for Neurology and Neurosurgery, Queen Square, London WC1N 3BG

Robert A H Surtees BM BCh PhD FRCP, Senior Lecturer in Paediatric Neurology, Institute of Child Health and Honorary Consultant Paediatric Neurologist, Great Ormond Street Hospital for Children, London WC1N 3JH

Wendy J Taylor MB ChB FRCR FRCP, Consultant Neuroradiologist, Hospital for Sick Children and National Hospital for Neurology and Neurosurgery, Queen Square, London WC1N 3BG

P K Thomas CBE MD DSc MRCS FRCP FRCPath, Emeritus Professor and Honorary Consultant, Royal Free Hospital School of Medicine, London NW3 2QG and National Hospital for Neurology and Neurosurgery, Queen Square, London WC1N 3BG, and Royal National Orthopaedic Hospital, London W1P 8AQ

Alan J Thompson MD FRCP FRCPI, Professor of Clinical Neurology and Rehabilitation, Department of Clinical Neurology, Institute of Neurology, Queen Square, London WC1N 3BG

Adrian J Wills MB BS MD MRCP, Locum Consultant Neurologist, King's College Hospital, London SE5 9RS

Nicholas W Wood MB ChB PhD MRCP, Senior Lecturer and Honorary Consultant Neurologist, National Hospital for Neurology and Neurosurgery, Queen Square, London WC1N 3BG

ix

PREFACE

The 'Grand Round' at Queen Square is an exciting weekly event. The wealth of clinical material passing through the National Hospital for Neurology and Neurosurgery provides three or four fascinating cases each week. Each patient's history is given, the physical signs are demonstrated, the differential diagnosis is discussed, and the investigations are presented. The occasion provides clinical vignettes of common and rare neurological conditions, with the usual complement of diagnostic dilemmas. Many clinicians who train at Queen Square comment that Thursday afternoon—the 'Grand Round'—is the highlight of the week, providing a memorable educational seminar. Dr Adrian Wills has captured the atmosphere of these traditional and classic occasions in *Fifty Neurological Cases from the National Hospital*. We hope it will provide enjoyment to those fascinated by clinical neurology.

CDM
London, July 1998

ACKNOWLEDGEMENTS

We are indebted to our colleagues, 30 neurologists and neurosurgeons, for their commentaries. Written from personal experience at Queen Square, as well as at other institutions, they have provided the reader with an immense amount of interpretation and knowledge. We are also grateful to our commissioning editor at Martin Dunitz Ltd, Alan Burgess. He and his colleague Susan Grant have ensured that an expeditious publishing schedule was maintained.

INTRODUCTION

There has been a 'Grand Round' at the National Hospital, Queen Square since it was opened in 1860 – so in a sense this is a book which has been waiting to be written for over a century. I claim no originality for the idea but I was blessed with enough time to write up the cases which had been presented during the year when I was Senior Registrar on the academic firm. I hope this book will appeal to neurologists at all stages of their careers. In addition, there are a number of clinical problems included which could provide a useful teaching aid to those candidates preparing for the MRCP. Each is presented in a traditional format so that the reader may attempt to formulate a differential diagnosis from the history and examination findings. I have been extremely fortunate in that established and emerging authorities in the field have commented on each case. Even the best clinicians occasionally suffer from diagnostic uncertainty and to reflect this fact I have also included a case which was originally discussed in 1877 and for which there is no definite solution. I am grateful to all the contributors who gave me unstintingly of their expertise. My special thanks go to the audio-visual department at the National who have provided most of the wonderful illustrations as well as to Professors MJG Harrison, WI McDonald, AJ Thompson, PN Leigh and Doctors N Wood, M Hanna, N Silver, JM Land and M Parton for permission to reproduce their slides. Finally, I would like to dedicate this book to my two children, Gabrielle and Fergus.

Adrian J Wills

CASE 1

History	A 71-year-old woman developed progressive facial weakness at the age of 20. Following this she presented with bloody diarrhoea necessitating a hemicolectomy. Twenty years later she began to complain of parasthaesiae, numbness and weakness involving her hands and feet. Her gait became ataxic and the facial weakness progressed, resulting in bilateral incomplete eyelid closure. At the age of 45 she complained of sudden visual loss affecting the left eye which was found later to be secondary to a central retinal vein occlusion complicated by rubeotic glaucoma. Visual function subsequently deteriorated in the right eye. At the age of 67 she had a stroke-like episode resulting in right sided weakness which resolved over the following month. Her two sisters, father, a paternal uncle and grandmother were affected by the same condition.

Examination

Visual acuity was reduced to finger counting on the right and light perception on the left. There was bilateral corneal scarring with lattice dystrophy. Fundi were normal. Impairment of ocular movements was compatible with an external ophthalmoplegia. Facial sensation was reduced and both corneal reflexes were absent. There was profound bilateral lower motor neurone facial weakness. The other cranial nerves were intact. Examination of the peripheral nervous system revealed pseudoathetosis with distal symmetrical weakness. Reflexes were intact and both plantar responses were extensor. Sensory examination revealed distal reduction of pinprick, temperature and light touch in a glove and stocking distribution. In addition, there was loss of joint position and vibration sense at the extremities. Her gait was ataxic.

Investigations

Routine blood tests, including liver, thyroid and renal function, were normal. MRI of the brain demonstrated evidence of a previous left middle cerebral artery occlusion. MRI of the cord was normal. Nerve conduction studies showed evidence of a mixed sensory–motor axonal neuropathy. An intestinal biopsy stained positively for amyloid. DNA analysis revealed the presence of an A-G mutation at position 654 of the gelsolin gene.

Diagnosis Finnish familial amyloid polyneuropathy

Commentary by Dr Mary M Reilly

In Finnish familial amyloid polyneuropathy (FAP) the constituent amyloidogenic protein is a mutated form of gelsolin so this form of amyloid is known as gelsolin-derived familial amyloid polyneuropathy. This type of FAP (type IV, old classification) was first noted in a Finnish kindred by Meretoja in 1969 but since then has been described in Holland, Japan, USA and the Czech Republic. Corneal lattice dystrophy often develops in the third or fourth decade, although this is often asymptomatic. This is followed by the insidious development of a progressive cranial neuropathy in the fifth or sixth decades. The facial nerve is commonly involved, with preponderant involvement of the upper fibres (Figure 1). Other cranial nerves that may be affected are the trigeminal, hypoglossal and vestibulocochlear nerves. The facial skin is thickened at first but with time it becomes lax. A mild sensory peripheral neuropathy may develop later. Autonomic involvement, if present, is mild.

The fibril protein in this disease is an abnormal fragment of gelsolin. There have been two point mutations in the gelsolin gene associated with this type of FAP; a substitution of asparagine for aspartic acid at residue 187 and a substitution of tyrosine for aspartic acid at the same position. The first mutation, Asn 187, which this patient had, has now been described in over 200 Finnish kindreds but has also been described in patients of Dutch, Japanese and Irish-American origins. A recent haplotype study has suggested an independent genetic origin for this mutation in Japan and Finland. The second gelsolin mutation, Tyr 187,

2

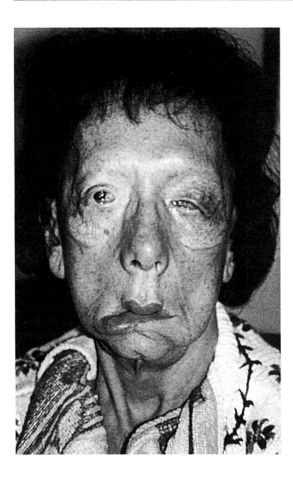

Figure 1 Finnish familial amyloid polyneuropathy (FAP). Characteristic facial appearance in a patient with FAP IV. Courtesy of Dr N Wood.

has been reported in only two families, one Danish and one Czech. The above patient is of particular interest as she is the first patient in Britain to be described with this disease. Haplotype studies will be of interest to see if they suggest a common ancestor with the Finnish families or an independent founder.

Reference

Reilly MM, Staunton H. Peripheral nerve amyloidosis. *Brain Pathol* 1996;**6**:163–77.

CASE 2

History   A 33-year-old man was well until the age of 19 when he
started having generalised tonic clonic seizures and
phenytoin was instituted. Six years later he developed
'absence' and 'drop' attacks with occasional myoclonic jerks.
Assessment at that stage revealed an ataxic gait and
carbamazepine was substituted for the phenytoin. His ataxia
continued to progress. The seizures were partially controlled
by a combination of lamotrigine and valproate. He was
retired on medical grounds at the age of 30 due to a
combination of increasing unsteadiness and cognitive
decline. The family history was negative and he did not
abuse alcohol.

Examination

The patient's higher mental functions were globally impaired. Cranial nerve
examination revealed abnormal eye movements with hypometric saccades,
saccadic intrusion into pursuit and square wave jerks. In the peripheral nervous
system there was a mixed movement disorder with dystonia and myoclonic jerks
(non-stimulus-sensitive). There were additional cerebellar signs consisting of
finger–nose and heel–shin ataxia, dysdiachokinesis and an ataxic gait. Tone,
power and reflexes were normal with flexor plantar responses. Sensory
examination was unremarkable.

Investigations

Psychometric testing revealed a performance IQ of 50 and a verbal IQ of 60.
The patient was rather disorientated and performed particularly poorly on tests
of memory. Routine haematology and biochemistry, including copper studies,
were normal. Blood films for acanthocytes were negative. Muscle and skin
biopsies were normal. Urinary organic and amino acids were normal. An EEG

5

showed generalised polyspike and wave discharges. MRI of the brain demonstrated generalised atrophy. Genetic studies were positive for the expanded trinucleotide (CAG) repeat in the DAPLA gene on chromosome 12.

Diagnosis   Dentatorubropallidoluysian atrophy (DRPLA)

Commentary by Dr Nicholas W Wood

DRPLA is a rare autosomal dominant disorder, which is more prevalent in Japan than in the western world. It has a variable clinical presentation and although there is overlap between the phenotypes they can essentially be grouped into three:

(i)   Presenting with chorea and dementia and resembling Huntington's disease (interestingly, another CAG repeat disease) but often with the additional feature of epilepsy;

(ii)   Ataxia as the predominant feature which may mimic a complicated autosomal dominant cerebellar ataxia (ADCA type 1);

(iii) Or as this case illustrates, presenting as a progressive myoclonic ataxia/epilepsy.

The disorder was mapped to a gene on chromosome 12p in Japan and the abnormality was shown to be an expanded CAG repeat. The normal range of CAG repeats varies between 6 and 35, whereas disease causing alleles vary from 54 to 80 plus repeats. At the time of writing this is one of eight disorders due to an expanded CAG, which encodes a polyglutamine tract (these include spinocerebellar ataxia (SCA)1,2,3,6 and 7-all autosomal dominant cerebellar ataxias, Kennedy's syndrome, Huntington's disease and DRPLA). Most of these disorders share some common features including cell specific neuronal degeneration, anticipation with greater instability in paternal transmissions and a positive correlation between repeat length and age of onset. It is probable that most (if not all) of these mutations are acting in a toxic gain of function manner. The precise mechanism of cell death remains unknown but it is clearly of great interest to scientific and neurological communities as it is hoped that there may well be a common downstream pathway for most of these disorders, and that a therapy may be designed upon this basis.

Reference

Nagafuchi S, Yanagiswa H, Sato K, *et al*. Dentatorubral and pallidoluysian atrophy, expansion of an unstable CAG trinucleotide on chromosome 12p. *Nature Genetics* 1994;**6**:14–18.

CASE 3

History   A 31-year-old man sustained a flexion–extension neck injury as a result of a judo throw. He was unconscious for several minutes and on recovery was noted to be quadraparetic. One week after the injury he developed blurred vision and was found to have significantly reduced visual acuity and failure of upgaze.

Examination

Visual acuity was reduced to finger counting in both eyes. Visual field testing indicated an inferior homonymous quadrantanopia. There was impairment of upgaze with impaired convergence and a brisk pupillary reaction to light. The patient had a quadraparesis which was far more marked in the upper than in the lower limbs. Power was 4+ (MRC scale) in the lower limbs and 3 at best in the upper limbs with a pyramidal pattern. Shoulder shrug was normal. Reflexes were pathologically brisk and plantar responses were extensor. He was catheterised. He had impairment of joint position sense in all four limbs which was far more marked in the arms than the legs. In addition he also had involvement of all other sensory modalities with a level to pinprick at C2/3.

Investigations

An MRI scan of the neck showed an avulsion fracture of the atlas with rupture of the transverse ligament. In addition, there was an intrinsic abnormal signal in the cord at C1/2 level and a more linear, less well defined lesion extending over a longer segment. There was no evidence of haemorrhage. MR angiography revealed patent vertebral arteries proximally. At the cephalad end of the right vertebral artery, just before its union with the left vertebral to form the basilar artery, the signal was attenuated secondary to poor blood flow consistent with a vertebral artery dissection. An MRI brain scan was normal.

> **Diagnosis** Traumatic high cervical cord injury with secondary vertebral artery dissection

Commentary by Mr H Alan Crockard

Injuries to the upper cervical spine and craniocervical junction are under diagnosed. Up to 40% of odontoid fractures are not detected at the time of injury either because they are unsuspected or because, as in this case, the injury can be ligamentous without any obvious bony abnormality on plain X-ray. Any patient complaining of neck or suboccipital pain after a flexion and extension road traffic or sporting injury should have very careful lateral flexion and extension plain radiographs to exclude a lesion. Moreover, patients who have been rendered transiently quadriparetic or had a short period of apnoea, particularly in the absence of a history of unconsciousness, have an injury at the craniovertebral junction until proven otherwise. Such patients should be very carefully evaluated, ideally with MRI in addition to plain X-rays. Vascular injuries associated with acute flexion and extension injuries of the neck are more commonly found in the carotid distribution and classically present several days after the injury with what are assumed to be platelet emboli. Non-fatal dissections of the vertebral arteries associated with injury are extremely rare. They are usually associated with a distracting mechanism of the head such as in the hanging type injury or, more frequently, where there has been an element of rotation causing an atlantoaxial rotatory subluxation or dislocation. While this latter injury is quite common and relatively benign in children, it is almost invariably fatal in adults. The interesting point in this man's history is that he survived without severe neurological deficit in the long term, despite a lesion that might have left him quadriplegic as a result of the primary injury or due to the problems that occurred a week later.

Reference

Thibodeaux LC, Hearn AT, Peschiera JL, *et al*. Extracranial vertebral artery dissection after trauma: a 5-year review. *Br J Surg* 1997;**84**:94–6.

CASE 4

History   A 34-year-old woman complained of lower limb weakness. As
a schoolgirl she had always been poor at sport and found it
difficult to keep up with her peers when walking. Her legs
were noted to be thin. She had difficulty getting shoes to fit
because her feet were high-arched. In her mid-twenties she
found it increasingly difficult to walk long distances without
tiring. Around the same time she noticed increasing cramps in
her calves. At the age of 30 she developed progressive
weakness of her hands. She also noticed increased fat
deposition over the face and underneath her chin. She found
that when dieting, her limbs would become thinner but her
trunk stayed the same size. Her alcohol consumption was low.

Examination

There were bilaterally symmetric deposits of body fat around the shoulder
girdle, neck, hips, thighs and thorax. The patient's gait was unsteady with
marked lower limb wasting and pes cavus. She was unable to stand on her heels.
Wasting of the triceps, brachioradialis and intrinsic hand muscles was noted.
Power in the upper limbs was relatively preserved proximally. There was
marked distal upper limb weakness. In the lower limbs, proximal power was
also relatively preserved. Reflexes were absent and both plantar responses were
flexor. There was a glove and stocking pattern of sensory loss involving light
touch and pinprick with preservation of joint position and vibration sense.

Investigations

Routine haematology and biochemistry were normal. Lactate level was normal.
Nerve conduction studies revealed evidence of a predominantly motor axonal
neuropathy. A muscle biopsy showed changes of chronic partial denervation. No
ragged red fibres were seen.

Diagnosis Madelung's disease

Commentary by Professor P K Thomas

Madelung's disease, or multiple symmetrica lipomatosis, is a disorder in which a spot diagnosis can be made readily (Figure 2). The bilaterally symmetric lipomata affecting the neck, trunk and proximal limbs are highly characteristic.

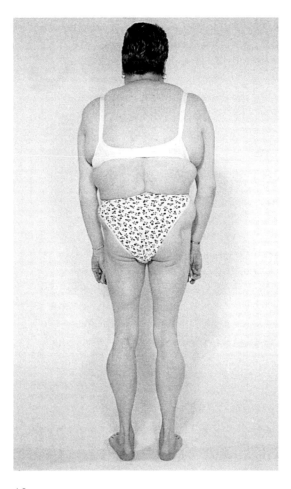

Figure 2 *Madelung's disease. Typical body habitus.*

The disorder is rare and of autosomal recessive inheritance. In a high proportion of patients there is a distal length-related symmetric and predominantly motor polyneuropathy. The age of presentation of the neuropathy is variable, the onset of symptoms either being delayed into adult life or commencing in childhood. In this patient the onset was early and insidious; her athletic prowess in school was restricted and the presence of pes cavus indicates that the neuropathy began before the cessation of the growth period. By her fourth decade she was severely handicapped. Electrophysiological and nerve biopsy studies have shown that the neuropathy is of axonal type. There is dispute as to whether this is associated with axonal atrophy, but there are no specific morphological features. Some patients show evidence of accompanying involvement of the central nervous system, including cerebellar ataxia. The basic metabolic defect in Madelung's disease is unknown. There have been recent reports of mitochondrial dysfunction in some cases but this was not evident in our patient. A fasting blood lactate level was normal and her muscle biopsy did not demonstrate the presence of ragged red fibres. It has been suggested that the neuropathy in Madelung's disease is related to alcohol abuse. This can be excluded in our patient as her neuropathy began in childhood and there was no indication of excessive alcohol consumption as an adult.

Reference

Klopstock T, Naumann M, Schalke B, *et al*. Multiple symmetric lipomatosis: abnormalities of complex IV and multiple deletions in mitochondrial DNA. *Neurology* 1994;**44**:862–6.

CASE 5

History   A 32-year-old man presented with a 3-month history of unsteadiness and poor coordination. He also complained of increasing irritability, poor concentration and memory. He did not abuse alcohol and was not receiving any treatment. There was no relevant family history. He had been treated for short stature 20 years earlier.

Examination

The patient had a wide based gait and performed heel–toe walking poorly. He was mildly dysarthric with a slight head tremor. He had dysmmetria in the upper limbs and minimal dysdiachokinesis. Coordination in the lower limbs was also affected. His eye movements were abnormal with saccadic intrusion into pursuit and square wave jerks. There was no myoclonus.

Investigations

Routine biochemistry and haematology were normal. An MRI brain scan was normal. EEG was normal. CSF analysis was normal apart from a raised protein level (0.8 g/l). Oligoclonal bands were negative.

Diagnosis   Iatrogenic Jakob–Creutzfeldt disease

Commentary by Dr Martin N Rossor

Most cases of Creutzfeldt–Jacob disease (CJD) or prion disease are sporadic: about 15% are familial and a small number are iatrogenic. Iatrogenic transfer has been reported with corneal transplants, neurosurgery (including depth electrodes) and cadaveric dura mater. Transmission by the use of cadaveric pituitary-derived growth hormone for treatment of small stature was first described in 1985. Nearly 2000 individuals have received this treatment in the United Kingdom and more than 10,000 in the United States. One hundred cases of iatrogenic CJD due to pituitary-derived growth hormone have now been recorded in the USA, UK and France. Four cases have been reported in Australia, linked to the use of pituitary-derived gonadotrophin. Whereas intracerebral and intraocular transmission results in a clinical picture more reminiscent of classical CJD (i.e. characterised by a rapidly progressive dementia), peripheral inoculation, as here, presents with a syndrome more akin to kuru. Thus there is a prolonged incubation period of around 15 years and a progressive ataxia with late cognitive change. There is a genetic susceptibility with an excess incidence reported in those with codon 129 homozygosity, in particular of the valine 129 allele. Definitive diagnosis depends upon histology and demonstration of prion protein immunoreactivity. The EEG is helpful in classical CJD, but less so in iatrogenic cases. Diagnostic aids that have been developed include the measurement of protein P14-3-3 in cerebrospinal fluid, although this is not specific. Recently, prion immunostaining has been demonstrated in tonsillar biopsy tissue. The diagnostic role of this latter method has yet to be established and experience is limited in iatrogenic CJD.

Reference

Collinge J. Human Prion Diseases: Aetiology and clinical features. In: Rossor MN, ed. *The Dementias.* Oxford: Butterworth-Heinemann, 1998.

CASE 6

History   A 40-year-old man presented with a 5-year history of constant high-pitched tinnitus in the left ear followed by hearing loss which progressed to involve the right ear. He also reported a 2-year history of gait ataxia and was unable to walk in a straight line. In addition, he developed symptoms suggestive of writers' cramp. His previous alcohol intake had exceeded 5 units per day. There was a family history of Ménière's disease.

Examination

The patient was ataxic and performed heel–toe walking poorly. He had dystonic posturing of the right hand both spontaneously and on attempting to write. Saccadic eye movements to target were abnormal with hypermetria and subsequent correction. Otherwise his eye movements were entirely normal. He had bilateral sensory neural hearing loss and a fine postural tremor. There was bilateral dysdiachokinesis and lower limb incoordination. In addition, he exhibited mild extrapyramidal slowing of finger movements of the right hand.

Investigations

Routine haematology and biochemistry, including iron studies, were normal. MRI of the brain showed marked haemosiderin deposition over the cerebellum, pons, midbrain and both thalami. The fourth, fifth and eighth cranial nerves were also affected bilaterally. The surface of the cerebral hemispheres was involved to a lesser extent. There was marked cerebellar atrophy. Cerebral angiography was normal.

Diagnosis   Haemosiderosis

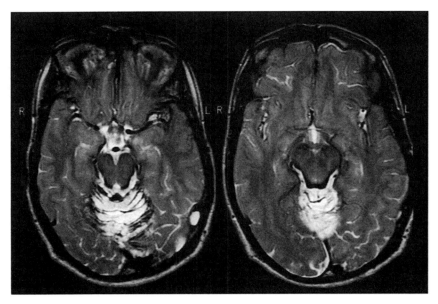

Figure 3 *Haemosiderosis. T2 weighted MRI scan demonstrating a thin dark rim around the surface of the brain stem and cerebellum.*

Commentary by Dr Peter Rudge

The history in this patient is typical of siderosis of the central nervous system, in which hearing loss and ataxia are the commonest two features. There have been no postmortem studies of the cochlea in these cases but the clinical presentation strongly suggests that the origin of the hearing deficit is the nerve fibre rather than something more peripheral. Characteristically, these patients have a speech audiogram that is much worse than expected from the pure tone audiometry findings. In addition, the stapedius reflexes have abnormal decay or are absent, there is no evidence of loudness recruitment and the brainstem evoked potentials are grossly abnormal. Furthermore, the cochlear emissions are normal. Pathologically, there is damage to the eighth nerve and MRI shows extensive deposition of iron along that nerve. Interestingly, the damage is confined to the centrally myelinated regions. The eighth nerve has a much greater proportion of its length occupied by oligodendrocytes than any other cranial nerve except the optic nerve. Somewhat counter-intuitively, cochlear

18

implants often help these patients appreciate speech. In adults, only a small proportion of cases have an obvious source of bleeding. It is noteworthy that some patients have evidence of nerve root avulsion in the cervical region, suggesting that varicosities in this area may be of aetiological relevance. MRI has revolutionised the diagnosis of this condition. T2 weighted images show clear signal void surrounding the affected areas (Figure 3). The superior cerebellum is particularly affected, presumably accounting for the associated ataxia. Unfortunately, if a bleeding point cannot be found, the prognosis is grave and most patients progress relentlessly. Trials of chelating agents have been disappointing. For this reason, it is vital that patients are investigated extensively to exclude any source of bleeding and angiography of the spinal cord and brain are mandatory.

Reference

Fearnley JM, Stevens JM, Rudge P. Superficial siderosis of the central nervous system. *Brain* 1995;**118:**1051–66.

CASE 7

History	A 53-year-old man developed flu-like symptoms 3 days after returning from holiday in Spain. His neck became swollen and he had a sore throat, with difficulty swallowing. He was noted to be pyrexial (38.5°C) with a tonsillar exudate and cervical lymphadenopathy. He was admitted to hospital and received a course of intravenous antibiotics. He made a full recovery. Five weeks later he complained of increasing dysphagia and noted that his voice had developed a nasal quality. As a consequence, a nasogastric tube was inserted. He then noticed difficulty walking with associated paraesthesiae affecting his lower extremities.

Examination

There was no evidence of ophthalmoplegia or ptosis. Pupillary reactions were normal. The patient's speech was nasal and palatal sensation and movement were reduced bilaterally. His uvula deviated to the right on phonation. Tongue movements were normal. There was a predominantly distal weakness in the limbs with tendon areflexia. Both plantar responses were flexor. Sensory examination revealed a glove and stocking loss to light touch and pinprick with lesser involvement of joint position and vibration sense. There was no nerve thickening or clinical evidence of autonomic dysfunction. General examination was unremarkable.

Investigations

Routine haematology and biochemistry were normal. Throat swabs and monospot were negative. CSF analysis was normal and negative for oligoclonal bands. Nerve conduction studies showed evidence of a demyelinating polyneuropathy. Antibody level to the diphtheria exotoxin was 0.5 units (normal range <0.1).

Diagnosis Diphtheritic polyneuropathy

Commentary by Professor P K Thomas

Diphtheria is now rare in western countries, although it is still prevalent in developing countries. Those who supervised the initial pharyngitis in this patient can therefore be excused for not recognising diphtheria, but the diagnosis clearly had to be considered when he developed a demyelinating polyneuropathy 5 weeks later. The differential diagnosis included the Guillain–Barré syndrome, but the combination of a predominantly motor neuropathy in the limbs with bulbar weakness made diphtheritic neuropathy highly probable. Interestingly, the patient did not show an iridocycloplegia and there was no evidence of cardiac involvement. The diagnosis was confirmed by the finding of elevated antibody levels to *Corynebacterium diphtheriae* exotoxin, indicating recent infection. The patient's mother could not recall whether he had been immunised against diphtheria in childhood. The exotoxin of *C. diphtheriae* produces a pure demyelinating neuropathy without inflammatory changes or axonal loss when administered experimentally in animals. This is the result of impaired synthesis of myelin basic protein. The exotoxin becomes fixed in the Schwann cells very rapidly after administration. The delay between the administration of the toxin, or the initiating infection in patients, and the onset of the neuropathy is related to the normal slow turnover of myelin. Recovery by remyelination is rapid and complete.

Reference

McDonald WI, Kocen RS, Diphtheritic neuropathy. In: Dyck PJ, Thomas PK, Griffin JW *et al*. Eds. *Peripheral Neuropathy* 3rd edn. Philadelphia: WB Saunders; 1993:1412–17.

CASE 8

History   A 56-year-old woman gave a 4-year history of progressive proximal lower limb weakness with associated tenderness of the thighs. A putative diagnosis of polymyositis was made and she was treated with steroids without benefit. She continued to deteriorate and her upper limbs became affected. In addition, she complained of mild dysphagia. Past medical and family history was non-contributory. She did not drink alcohol to excess.

Examination

The cranial nerves were normal with no evidence of ophthalmoplegia. Neck flexion was weak. Examination of the upper and lower limbs revealed proximal weakness and wasting. There was additional weakness of the flexor digitorum profundus in the upper limbs. Reflexes were normal and sensory examination was unremarkable. Plantar responses were flexor. Muscles were non-tender and there were no stigmata of a vasculitis or a connective tissue disorder.

Investigations

Routine haematology and biochemistry were normal. Thyroid function tests and creatine kinase levels were normal. Autoimmune profile, including anti-Jo 1 antibodies and ANCA were negative. An EMG revealed myopathic changes. A muscle biopsy showed marked abnormalities. There were rimmed vacuoles (Figure 4), intracellular amyloid deposits and an endomysial inflammatory infiltrate (Figure 5). Electron microscopy revealed cytoplasmic and nuclear tubulofilaments measuring 15 nm in diameter.

Diagnosis   Inclusion body myositis

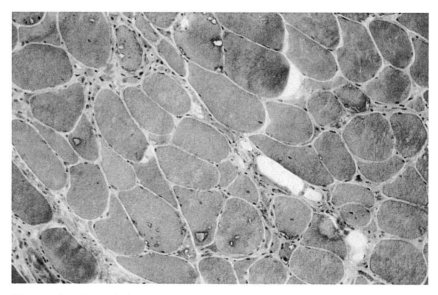

Figure 4 *Inclusion body myositis (IBM). Muscle biopsy showing rimmed vacuoles (Gomori trichrome stain). Courtesy of Dr M G Hanna.*

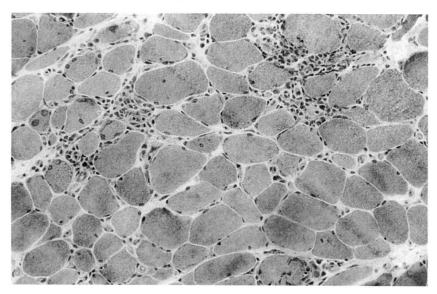

Figure 5 *Inclusion body myositis. Muscle biopsy demonstrating a marked inflammatory infiltrate (Gomori trichrome stain). Courtesy of Dr M G Hanna.*

Commentary by Dr Michael G Hanna

The history and examination in this 56-year-old woman clearly point to a myopathic process. The patient's age, particular involvement of the flexor digitorum profundus, dysphagia and lack of response to steroids all point to inclusion body myositis (IBM) but this remains a histopathological diagnosis. IBM is an idiopathic inflammatory myopathy which commonly develops between the ages of 50 and 70 years. Characteristically there is a symmetrical, steadily progressive muscle weakness involving all four limbs. The distribution varies and can be generalised, proximal or distal. In some cases there is particular involvement of the finger and wrist flexor muscles with relative preservation of the extensor muscles. Atrophy of the volar forearm muscles is also seen. In the lower limbs, the quadriceps femoris may be particularly affected. Atrophy of the affected muscles is frequent and proportionate to the degree of weakness. Cervical, facial and bulbar muscles may be involved but rarely to a severe extent. Mild dysphagia occurs in one-third of cases. The extraocular muscles are spared but respiratory muscle involvement occurs in 10% of cases. Transient myalgias are noted occasionally at the beginning or during the evolution of the illness. No association with malignancy has been documented but there is an association with some immune mediated disorders such as systemic lupus erythematosus, Sjögren's syndrome and diabetes mellitus. The ESR is typically normal and the CK may be normal or elevated less than ten-fold. As in other inflammatory myopathies, the EMG pattern can be neurogenic, myopathic or show a combination of the two. An accurate diagnosis relies on the muscle biopsy findings. The combination of rimmed vacuoles, an endomysial inflammatory infiltrate and intracellular amyloid deposits or filamentous inclusions seen on electron microscopy is said to be diagnostic. Groups of atrophic fibres may also be seen. The aetiology of IBM is unknown but there is a general view that it represents a degenerative disorder of skeletal muscle. The disease progresses relentlessly. Typically, patients remain ambulatory for many years after the onset of symptoms but they are eventually confined to a wheelchair. The available evidence suggests that most patients do not respond to immunotherapy such as steroids or intravenous immunoglobulins. There may be a small subgroup which does benefit from steroids.

Reference

Griggs RC, Askanas V, DiMauro S, et al. Inclusion body myositis and myopathies. *Ann Neurol* 1995;**38**:705–13.

CASE 9

History   A 64-year-old man had a history of leg cramps which developed 20 years previously. At the age of 50 he noticed progressive difficulty in getting out of a chair or climbing stairs. Following this, he developed proximal upper limb weakness. He noticed increasing dysphagia and was woken frequently by episodes of breathlessness. His wife reported that he had begun to snore loudly. There was no relevant family history. He did not drink alcohol to excess.

Examination

The patient had bilateral gynaecomastia. Cranial nerve examination revealed bilateral facial weakness. The jaw jerk was absent. His tongue was fasciculating and mildly wasted. Neck flexor muscles were weak. Examination of the limbs revealed mainly proximal wasting and fasciculation with corresponding weakness. The tone was normal, reflexes were absent and plantar responses were flexor. Sensory examination was unremarkable. Vital capacity was 1.6 litres standing and 0.8 litres lying. There was no evidence of paradoxical abdominal movements.

Investigations

Creatine kinase levels were normal. Glucose levels were normal. EMG studies showed evidence of denervation and renervation consistent with a chronic anterior horn cell disorder. DNA analysis revealed an expanded 50-length CAG triple repeat (normal range <27) in the androgen receptor gene.

Diagnosis   X-linked bulbospinal neuronopathy (Kennedy's syndrome)

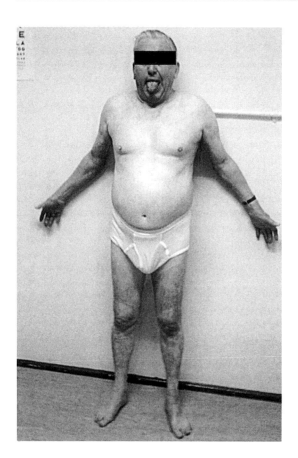

Figure 6 Kennedy's syndrome. Gynaecomastia and typical body habitus. Courtesy of Professor PN Leigh and Dr M Parton.

Commentary by Dr Nicholas W Wood

X-linked bulbospinal neuronopathy (XLBSN) was first described in the English speaking literature in 1966, by Kennedy and colleagues. The gene, as the name suggests, lies on the X chromosome and is inherited in a recessive manner. Onset of weakness is most commonly in the third and fourth decades but, as in this case, it can be later. The history described above is otherwise fairly typical, with a long history of leg cramps, before the development of definitive weakness, most frequently proximally, followed by atrophy in the lower extremities. The fasciculations and the bulbar atrophy may suggest the possibility of amyotrophic lateral sclerosis, but the length of history and associated features usually alerts the clinician to perform the definitive genetic test. Associated features include a characteristic hand tremor, non-insulin-dependent diabetes, infertility and gynaecomastia (Figure 6). The rate of progression is slow and patients usually remain ambulant until late in the course of disease. In 1991 the trinucleotide repeat CAG was found in exon 1 of the androgen receptor gene. This was the first of what has become a growing family of CAG triplet repeat disorders. In all of these disorders, an expansion of a CAG tract (CAG encodes glutamine) within the coding region of a gene gives rise to a neurodegenerative condition. The nature of the disease depends upon the gene in which the polyglutamine tract is located. The normal range of triplet repeats is usually less than 34, whereas abnormal is defined as greater than 40. However, there is a grey area between 34 and 40, in which repeats may represent an intermediate or pre-mutation phase. Identification of cases is not only important in diagnostic terms but also in genetic counselling, in particular in the case of daughters of affected males, whose sons will have a 50% chance of being affected.

Reference

La Spada AR, Wilson EM, Lubhan DB, Harding AE, Fischbeck KH. Androgen receptor gene mutations in X-linked and bulbar spinal muscular atrophy. *Nature* 1991;**352**:77–9.

CASE 10

Examination

The patient had a stiff gait with an exaggerated lumbar lordosis. Her paraspinal muscles were extremely rigid. Cranial nerve and upper limb examination was normal. In the lower limbs, tone was increased. Power was full and reflexes were pathologically brisk. Both plantar responses were flexor. There were no sensory abnormalities and no evidence of myoclonus.

Investigations

Routine haematology and biochemistry were normal. Thyroid function tests were normal. Gastric parietal cell, intrinsic factor and anti-GAD antibodies were positive. Anti-islet cell antibodies were negative. Oligoclonal bands were present in serum and CSF with a matched pattern. MRI of the brain and spinal cord was normal. Nerve conduction studies were normal. An EMG showed continuous motor unit activity in the paraspinal muscles and vasti.

Diagnosis   Stiff person syndrome

Commentary by Dr Peter Brown

The stiff person syndrome was first described by Moersch and Woltmann in 1956. This is a chronic condition involving painful stiffness and spasm of the axial muscles. Spasms may be spontaneous or precipitated by voluntary action or unexpected 'startling' stimuli. As in the case presented, there is often a strong personal and family history of autoimmune disease, particularly insulin-dependent diabetes mellitus which is present in about one-third of cases. Investigations are important to exclude alternative diagnoses, particularly structural lesions of the cord, inflammatory conditions such as progressive encephalomyelitis with rigidity (which itself often has a paraneoplastic aetiology) or neuromyotonia. Thus, importantly in this case, MRI of the brain and spinal cord was normal, EMG studies confirmed continuous motor unit activity in axial muscles but furnished no evidence of neuromyotonia and CSF showed no increase in inflammatory cells. The presence of antibodies directed against glutamic acid decarboxylase (GAD) is helpful in confirming the diagnosis. Such antibodies are present in around 60% of most series. Oligoclonal bands are also commonly found in the CSF. The prognosis is generally good and most patients have an excellent response to combined therapy with oral diazepam and baclofen, often in high dosage. Resistant cases may be successfully treated with intrathecal Baclofen or parenteral immunoglobulins. The presence of anti-GAD antibodies, the association with autoimmune diseases and the response to pooled immunoglobulins suggest an autoimmune aetiology for the stiff person syndrome. The histological appearance of the brain and spinal cord is unremarkable in classical cases.

Reference

Lorish TR, Thorsteinsson G, Howard FM. Stiff man syndrome updated. *Mayo Clin Proc* 1989;**64**:629–36.

CASE 11

History	A 28-year-old alcoholic was admitted to hospital following acute ethanol intoxication. He was initially comatose but recovered fully and was discharged on a combination of thiamine and chlordiazepoxide. He was readmitted 10 days later with a 48-hour history of ataxia, tremor, dysarthria and dysphagia. Examination at that stage revealed him to be pyrexial and tremulous. He was ataxic but orientated in time and place. He was treated with intravenous fluids and vitamins. In spite of this, he developed increased tone in the limbs with pathologically brisk reflexes and a coarse nystagmus. His respiratory function deteriorated and he required ventilation.

Examination

The patient was ventilated but alert and extremely tearful. His vertical eye movements were normal but he developed pronounced nystagmus on attempted horizontal movement. He had a pyramidal increase in tone affecting all four limbs with grade 2 power in the upper limbs and grade 1 in the lower limbs. Reflexes were pathologically brisk with bilaterally extensor plantar responses and sustained clonus at both ankles.

Investigations

Initial biochemical and haematological screening was normal apart from hyponatraemia (Na-127 mmol/l), mildly raised ALT and γGT and macrocytosis (100 fl). CSF examination was normal. An EEG showed generalised slow waves. An MRI of the brain revealed hyperintense signal change on T2 weighting in the dorsal pons and in the region of the thalamic nuclei.

> **Diagnosis** Central pontine myelinolysis

Commentary by Professor Alan J Thompson

Central pontine myelinolysis (CPM), first described in a classic paper by Adams, Victor and Mancall in 1959, is seen particularly in the context of alcoholism and malnutrition. Other causes include Wilson's disease, burns and various malignancies. Virtually all cases have occurred in a hospital setting. Symmetrical myelin destruction of the basis pontis occurs with occasional extension into the pontine tegmentum. In 10% of cases the lesions lie outside the pons, usually affecting the thalamus or cerebellum. The classical clinical presentation is of a

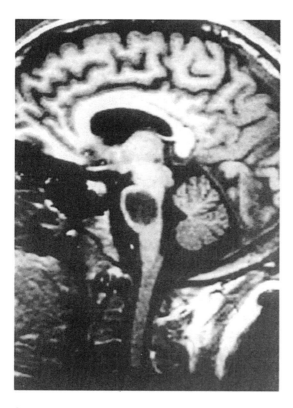

Figure 7 *Central pontine myelinolysis. T1 weighted MRI scan showing low density change in the mid pons. Courtesy of Professor AJ Thompson and Dr N Silver.*

rapidly evolving quadriparesis, pseudobulbar palsy and diminished level of consciousness with minimal sensory involvement. A locked-in syndrome may also occur. The condition is characterised pathologically by relative axonal sparing. It has been noted that transverse fibres tend to be more affected than longitudinal corticospinal fibres and this has been demonstrated on MRI with relative sparing of the ventral aspect of the pons (Figure 7). In the majority of cases, the mechanism of demyelination is thought to relate to rapid changes in sodium levels, frequently due to over energetic treatment of hyponatraemia. CPM may not always cause neurological dysfunction and may be an incidental finding at post mortem. However, when it causes a severe quadriplegia as described in this case, the outcome is usually fatal with a quoted survival rate of only 10%. Fortunately, our patient made a slow and steady recovery and returned to his pre-morbid state in 6 months.

Reference

Laureno R. Central pontine myelinolysis following rapid correction of hyponatraemia. *Ann Neurol* 1983;**13**:232–42.

CASE 12

History   A 33-year-old woman had normal early milestones and was good at sport when at school. At the age of 12 years she noticed stiffness of both calves after physical exertion. Her parents commented that her calves looked very 'muscular'. Four years later she noticed difficulty running and by the age of 18 years her gait was described as waddling. From the age of 26 years she began to complain of upper limb weakness. Within 2 years she was walking with the aid of two sticks. She had no dysphagia and no history suggestive of myoglobinuria. The family history was non-contributory.

Examination

Cranial nerve examination was normal with no evidence of ophthalmoplegia, facial weakness or retinopathy. Neck flexion and extension was normal. Examination of the limbs revealed global wasting with predominantly proximal weakness. There were no fasciculations. The patient was arreflexic and there were no sensory abnormalities. Beevor's sign was positive. She walked with a waddling gait and demonstrated Gower's manoeuvre on attempting to rise from a seated position.

Investigations

Creatine kinase was elevated at 3000 IU/l. EMG showed evidence of a chronic myopathic process with little spontaneous activity. A muscle biopsy was abnormal with an increase in connective tissue and marked variability in fibre diameter. There were scattered basophilic fibres suggestive of regeneration but no inflammatory infiltration. Staining for dystrophin and three components of the sarcoglycan complex were normal.

Diagnosis   Limb girdle muscular dystrophy

Commentary by Dr John A Morgan-Hughes

The autosomal recessive limb girdle muscular dystrophies (ARLGMD) are a clinically and genetically heterogeneous group of diseases which present in childhood or adult life with slowly progressive wasting and weakness of the proximal limb muscles with sparing of the face and usually of the neck flexor muscles. There may be hypertrophy of the calves and pseudohypertrophy of other muscles including the quadriceps femoris. Progression is variable, with some patients becoming wheelchair-bound in the second or third decades and others remaining ambulant until much later in life. The serum creatine kinase level is elevated 10 to 20 times the upper limit of normal. The EMG is myopathic and a muscle biopsy typically shows hypertrophied fibres, internal nucleation and proliferation of endomysial connective tissue with occasional myonecrosis. Progress in molecular genetics has heralded a new classification of the LGMDs based on the genes and gene products that are defective. ARLGMDs types 2C, 2D, 2E and 2F arise from mutations in the γ, α, β and δ sarcoglycan genes located at 13q12, 17q12–21.33, 4q12 and 5q33–q44 respectively and are now referred to as the sarcoglycanopathies. The four sarcoglycans identified to date are muscle-specific integral membrane components of the dystrophin–glycoprotein complex within the sarcolemma. ARLGMD type 2A arises from a mutation in the calpain 3 gene located at 15q15.1–q21.1 and ARLGMD type 2G has been mapped to 17q11–q12 but the gene product has not yet been identified. Classification of the LGMDs is likely to extend considerably as new mutations and their gene products are identified.

Reference

Campbell KP. The sarcoglycanopathies and related disorders. *Curr Opin Neurol* 1998 (In Press).

CASE 13

<table>
<tr>
<td>History</td>
<td>A 21-year-old man had developed a thoracic scoliosis 11 years previously. This had progressed and at the age of 14 years he underwent surgery with placement of Harrington rods. At the age of 19 years he developed gait ataxia, his hands became clumsy and his speech slurred. He was described as 'fidgety' by his parents and found it difficult to sit still. The family history was non-contributory.</td>
</tr>
</table>

Examination

Cognition was normal. The patient had generalised choreiform movements involving his face, trunk and limbs. There was no true gait ataxia. Cranial nerve examination was unremarkable apart from a mild slurring dysarthria. Eye movements were normal. Examination of the limbs revealed normal tone and power. Reflexes were absent and plantar responses were flexor. There were no sensory abnormalities.

Investigations

Routine haematology and biochemistry were normal. Vitamin E levels were normal, and there were no acanthocytes. CSF examination was normal. ECG was normal. Nerve conduction studies showed evidence of an axonal mainly sensory neuropathy. Genetic testing for SCA 1, 2, 3 and DRPLA was negative. However there was an expansion in the frataxin gene on chromosome 9.

<table>
<tr>
<td>Diagnosis</td>
<td>Friedreich's ataxia</td>
</tr>
</table>

Commentary by Dr Nicholas W Wood

Friedreich's ataxia is the most common of the hereditary ataxias with a prevalence of about 1 in 50,000. In addition to progressive gait and limb ataxia, the core features include absent reflexes, development of pyramidal signs within the first 5 years of illness, and frequently skeletal deformities (scoliosis and pes cavus). Additional supportive features include cardiomyopathy, which is most easily picked up with ECG (although subtle cases may need echocardiography), dysarthria, deafness, diabetes mellitus, and optic atrophy. The identification of the gene in early 1996 permitted a re-evaluation of the classical signs and a slight broadening of the phenotype, which includes a later age of onset (one case developed ataxia at 51 years old), retention of reflexes, pseudodominant inheritance and, as this case illustrates, choreiform movements. The genetic abnormality (in approximately 97% of cases) is an expanded GAA triplet repeat in intron 1 of the frataxin gene (the normal range is up to 50 repeats). In the remaining cases, compound heterozygosity has been demonstrated with a point mutation on an allele and an expansion on the other. Disease is associated with repeat lengths of greater than 200 and often more than 1000. This test is now widely available, and therefore should be performed on not only all classical cases of Friedreich's ataxia, but also suspected cases. The clinical clue in this patient was the presence of scoliosis associated with absent reflexes. It is likely that ataxia will develop with progression of the disease.

Reference

Harding AE. The inherited ataxias. *Adv Neurol* 1988;**48**:37–46.

CASE 14

History — A 15-year-old girl whose parents were consanguinous was the youngest of six siblings. Her initial milestones were entirely normal. At the age of 3 years she developed a stammer followed by behavioural problems and anorexia. She was noted to repetitively clap her hands. By the age of 6 years she began to show evidence of intellectual regression. She became increasingly dysarthric, immobile and incontinent of urine. By the age of 14 years she was unable to recognise other members of her family.

Examination

The patient was uncooperative and cried continuously. Her fundi and eye movements seemed normal. She had marked facial grimacing and facial dystonia. She exhibited purposeless flailing of the right arm with dystonic posturing of the left arm. Power was normal. Reflexes were symmetrically brisk with flexor plantar responses. There was no evidence of organomegaly.

Investigations

Routine haematology and biochemistry were normal. Analysis of white cell enzymes revealed hexosaminidase deficiency (0.2 micro-units, normal range 0.58–3.0 micro-units). This was confirmed by subsequent demonstration of hexosaminidase A and B deficiency in skin fibroblasts (90 units; normal range >10,000 units).

Diagnosis GM$_2$ gangliosidosis (Sandhoff disease)

Commentary by Dr Robert A H Surtees

GM_2 gangliosidosis is caused by deficiency or reduced activity of hexosaminidase A (Tay–Sachs disease) or A and B (Sandhoff disease), or rarely by deficiency of hexosaminidase activator protein. This leads to accumulation of GM_2 ganglioside, predominantly in the brain. Normally this is a disorder of early infancy with onset before 6 months of age and death before 4 years. In retrospect, the first symptom is an exaggerated startle response followed rapidly by blindness (optic atrophy and accumulation of ganglioside at the macula to give the characteristic cherry-red spot) and generalised spasticity. The infant develops dementia, losing all developmental skills, and seizures. In the late stages of the disease macrocephaly may develop. There is no effective treatment. Rarely, GM_2 gangliosidosis has a delayed onset. Juvenile GM_2 gangliosidosis has an onset after 3 years of age and the initial symptom is often a stutter which may have a dystonic component. Progressive gait disturbance (ataxic–spastic, occasionally with lower motor neurone involvement), dementia and seizures then develop. More rarely still, GM_2 gangliosidosis can present in adults with a spinocerebellar syndrome resembling Friedreich's ataxia or a clinical picture resembling motor neurone disease. Imaging may reveal diffuse cortical atrophy, white matter disease or thalamic hyperdensity presumed secondary to calcification.

Reference

Navon R. Molecular and clinical heterogeneity of adult GM_2 gangliosidosis. *Dev Neurosci* 1991;**13**:295–8.

CASE 15

History   A 33-year-old man noticed 5 years previously that he suffered increasing unsteadiness after drinking alcohol. His gait gradually deteriorated secondary to lower limb weakness. He became unable to run. He also complained of urinary urgency which had been present for a similar period of time. His upper limbs were unaffected. He had previously been fit and well and there was no family history of neurological or endocrine disorders.

Examination

The patient's gait was unsteady. Romberg's test was negative. There was no evidence of cognitive impairment. Cranial nerve examination was normal with no fundal abnormalities or ophthalmoplegia. The jaw jerk was normal. There were no upper limb abnormalities. In the lower limbs there was a spastic paraparesis with bilateral sustained ankle clonus and extensor plantar responses. The lower abdominal reflexes were absent. Upper limb reflexes were brisk but the lower limb reflexes were normal. There was mild distal impairment of vibration and joint position sense in the lower limbs. There was evidence of bilateral stocking sensory loss to light touch and pinprick.

Investigations

Routine haematology, including B_{12} levels, and biochemistry were normal. Treponemal serology was negative. Random cortisol was normal. A short synacthen test was abnormal (baseline cortisol 201 nmol/l rising to 274 nmol/l and 282 nmol/l after 30 and 60 minutes). Analysis of very long chain fatty acids revealed a raised C24/22 ratio (1.25; normal range <0.096) and a raised C26/22 ratio (0.044; normal range <0.022). CSF analysis was normal with negative oligoclonal bands. Nerve conduction studies were normal. MRI of the brain showed increased signal on T2 weighting around the posterior horns of the

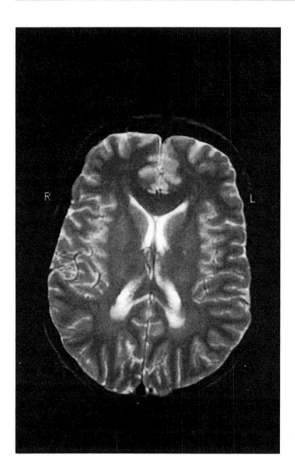

Figure 8 T2 weighted MRI scan demonstrating posterior white matter signal abnormalities.

lateral ventricles and in the region of the right middle cerebellar peduncle. MRI of the spine showed cord thinning with diffuse signal change in the thoracic region.

Diagnosis Adrenoleukodystrophy

Commentary by Professor David H Miller

Adrenoleukodystrophy (ALD) is an X-linked disease. It usually presents in boys as a relentlessly progressive leukodystrophy of cerebral hemisphere white matter resulting in severe behavioural and cognitive deficits within a few years. These changes often start in the posterior hemispheres and then move forwards. Presentation in adult males is not uncommon. This is usually as an isolated, slowly progressive spastic paraparesis (adrenomyeloneuropathy). A similar presentation may also occur in heterozygous adult females. As in this case, there may be evidence for hypoadrenalism in laboratory tests, and there may also be clinical concomitants including hyperpigmentation. A positive family history may be an important diagnostic clue. The key investigation is measurement of serum very long chain fatty acids (VLCFA), which are elevated. Almost all boys with the cerebral form of ALD have extensive MRI abnormalities, and gadolinium enhancement of the advancing edge of the lesion is characteristic. MRI in adults may be normal, or may show symmetrical cerebral white matter changes especially posteriorly, although this is less marked than in the childhood forms (Figure 8). Dietary supplementation with glyceryl trioleate and trierucate corrects the VLCFA abnormalities but does not appear to modify the disease course in those patients who are symptomatic. Whether this mode of therapy has a potential for delaying disease onset in ALD is currently being evaluated in a trial of asymptomatic children. Some authorities advocate bone marrow transplantation in children with MRI and neuropsychological abnormalities but no symptoms.

Reference

Moser HW. Adrenoleukodystrophy: phenotype, genetics, pathogenesis and therapy. *Brain* 1997;**120**:1485–1508.

CASE 16

History	A 24-year-old woman had normal developmental milestones. At the age of 10 years her school performance declined and her intellectual progress continued to cause her parents concern until she left school. In her teenage years she was said to be clumsy but was able to partake in sporting activities. At the age of 21 years she developed slurred speech. In the following year she became pregnant and it was noted that her speech and balance deteriorated. In addition, she developed emotional lability. She was otherwise well and there was no family history of neurological disorders. She was a non-smoker and did not abuse alcohol.

Examination

The patient scored 22/30 on the Mini Mental State Exam. She had particular difficulties with recall and exhibited dyscalculia. Her gait was ataxic and Romberg's test was negative. Cranial nerve examination revealed abnormalities of saccadic eye movements with particularly poor initiation of downgaze and reduced velocity. Pursuit eye movements were normal. The doll's eye manoeuvre was normal. Her tongue movements were slow with associated dysarthria. In the peripheral nervous system she exhibited evidence of dystonia and myoclonus especially affecting the upper limbs. Tone and power were normal and plantar responses were downgoing. There was no reflex asymmetry and no abnormalities of cutaneous sensation. General examination revealed a palpable splenic tip.

Investigations

Routine biochemistry and haematology were normal. White cell enzymes were normal and there was no evidence of acanthocytes. Copper studies were normal. Very long chain fatty acid levels were normal. Serum lactate was normal. Urinary organic and amino acids were normal. EEG showed no evidence of epileptiform activity or periodic complexes. EMG and nerve conduction studies were normal. An abdominal ultrasound confirmed splenic enlargement. MRI of the brain showed a bilateral diffuse increase in deep white matter signal on T2 weighting. Bone marrow aspiration revealed clear evidence of foamy irregular vacuoles and cellular debris.

Diagnosis   Niemann–Pick syndrome type C

Commentary by Dr Charles A Davie

Niemann–Pick syndrome is a heterogeneous condition with autosomal recessive inheritance. A number of subtypes have been recognised. These include an acute neuronopathic form (type A), a chronic form without nervous system involvement (type B), a chronic neuronopathic form (type C), Nova Scotia variant (type D), an adult non-neuronopathic form (type E), and a benign visceral form (type F). These phenotypes can also be alternatively classified into type I lipidosis where sphingomyelinase deficiency leads to sphingomyelin accumulation in all tissues, and type II lipidosis where the primary defect is uncertain and a secondary partial reduction of sphingomyelin activity results. Niemann–Pick type C (NPC) forms part of the latter group and is a neurovisceral disorder characterised by lysosomal accumulation of low density lipoprotein (LDL) derived cholesterol. A gene (NPC1) has been identified on chromosome 18q which seems to be partly responsible for the dysregulation of cholesterol trafficking in this condition. The clinical features of NPC include organomegaly, psychomotor regression, ataxia, vertical gaze palsy, dystonia, macular cherry red spot, seizures, developmental delay, a demyelinating polyneuropathy and pyramidal signs. Sea-blue histiocytes and foam cells are seen in the bone marrow in most cases but are not specific (Figure 9).

The combination of ataxia, cognitive decline and a supranuclear vertical gaze palsy, as seen in our case, is strongly suggestive of NPC. Other conditions to be excluded in this context include Wilson's disease, Gaucher's disease (in which the gaze palsy tends to be horizontal rather than vertical), GM_2 gangliosidosis,

48

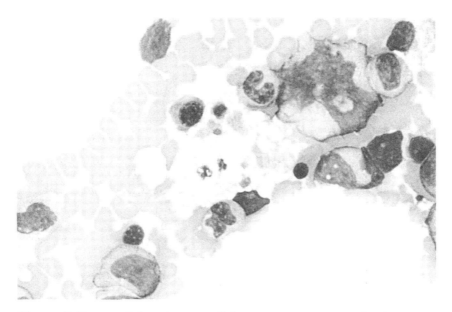

Figure 9 *Niemann–Pick syndrome type C. Bone marrow aspirate stained with May–Grünwald Giemsa. Numerous foamy storage cells are visible. The presence of debris and irregular vacuolation are characteristic. Courtesy of Professor B Lake.*

ataxia–telangiectasia and Whipple's disease, which may be entirely confined to the nervous system. New variant Creutzfeldt–Jakob disease should also be considered in a young adult with recent cognitive decline. These patients may also have evidence of an upgaze palsy. Other genetic disorders which may present similarly include Huntington's disease, dentatorubropallidoluysian atrophy, and the SCA2 genotype of autosomal dominant cerebellar ataxia (type I) in which there is marked slowing of saccadic eye movements. These last three conditions, which are all transmitted in autosomal dominant fashion, are examples of a CAG polyglutamine tract repeat disorder and can be diagnosed by appropriate genetic testing. Attempts to reduce cholesterol synthesis or LDL formation in NPC have been ineffective in altering the disease progression. However, the identification of a human gene, together with the identification of a cholesterol homeostasis gene in a mouse model of NPC, will hopefully lead to new therapeutic strategies in future.

Reference

Carstea ED, Morris JA, Coleman KG, *et al.* Niemann–Pick C1 disease gene: homology to mediators of cholesterol homeostasis. *Science* 1997;**277:**228–31.

CASE 17

History	A 20-year-old right-handed woman had presented 3 years previously with colicky abdominal pain and bloody diarrhoea. A small bowel biopsy was diagnostic of Crohn's disease and she was given treatment with mesalazine which led to marked symptomatic improvement. Three months prior to admission her abdominal symptoms recurred and she was treated with oral steroids. Following this, she developed a sore throat requiring antibiotic therapy. She remained in bed for 3 days, following which she developed a gradual onset of frontotemporal headache with associated right upper limb weakness and numbness. Her speech became dysphasic and on the day of admission she had a right-sided focal motor seizure with secondary generalisation.

Examination

The patient was apyrexial and drowsy (post-ictally) with no neck stiffness. There was no papilloedema. She had a mild expressive dysphasia and a right homonymous hemianopia. There was evidence of a mild right pyramidal weakness and right-sided sensory inattention. The right plantar response was extensor.

Investigations

Results are shown in Table 1. Liver function tests were normal, apart from mild elevation of ALP and γGT. Autoimmune profile including ANCA was negative. Clotting screen, including protein C and S, antithrombin III and lupus anticoagulant was negative, as were blood cultures. Folate levels were normal. CSF analysis revealed an opening pressure of 23 cm. Oligoclonal bands were positive in serum and CSF. A CT scan of the brain showed clear evidence of the

Table I Haematological and biochemical investigations	
haemoglobin	8.0 g/dl (normochromic, normocytic)
ESR	80 mm/h
platelets	$800 \times 10^9/l$
white cell count	$9.0 \times 10^9/l$
CRP	106 mg/l
albumin	25 g/l
vitamin B_{12}	187 ng/l (normal = 223–1132 ng/l)
CSF protein	0.67 g/l
CSF white cell count	<1
CSF glucose	normal

'delta sign' (Figure 10). An MRI scan of the brain confirmed the presence of thrombosis in the superior, straight and right transverse sinuses.

Diagnosis   Crohn's disease complicated by venous sinus thrombosis

---

Commentary by Dr Adrian J Wills

Crohn's disease is an idiopathic intestinal disorder of unknown cause. It has been postulated that increased platelet activation leading to multifocal microinfarction in the mesenteric vasculature may be the primary pathogenic event in this illness. In addition, there is evidence that associated disorders of factors V and VIII and fibrinogen with decreased levels of antithrombin III may contribute to the resultant hypercoagulable state. This may explain the observation that thromboembolic events are relatively common in patients with Crohn's disease. Alternative explanations for the increased incidence of thromboembolism include the presence of circulating immune complexes as a consequence of vasculitis, associated autoantibodies (including ANCA) and antiphospholipid antibodies or prolonged dehydration and immobilisation secondary to active

52

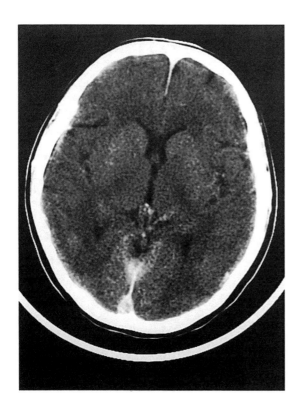

Figure 10 *Venous sinus thrombosis. Contrast enhanced CT scan demonstrating the 'delta' sign (enhancement around a clot in the saggital sinus).*

disease. Cerebral arterial and venous events have been described and tend to occur when the illness is active, as in this case. Cerebral arterial occlusions occur in larger vessels in both anterior and posterior territories. Venous thrombosis may lead to secondary haemorrhagic infarction. Most experts agree that the treatment of uncomplicated venous sinus thrombosis includes anticoagulation. However, if the underlying Crohn's disease is active this obviously increases the risk of severe gastrointestinal haemorrhage and management decisions should involve close cooperation between the neurologist and gastroenterologist.

Reference

Wills AJ, Hovell CJ. Neurological complications of enteric disease. *Gut* 1996;**39**:501–4.

CASE 18

History   A 39-year-old woman developed intermittent stiffness and
weakness of the legs 1 year before presentation. She had
particular difficulty climbing stairs. A striking feature of her
illness was the close temporal association of her symptoms
and the menstrual cycle. Over the next year the symptoms
became continuous between catamenial exacerbations. The
patient developed urinary frequency and occasional urge
incontinence with associated constipation. She was found to
have a raised titre of antinuclear antibodies with
thrombocytopaenia (platelets $100 \times 10^9/l$) and a mild
lymphopaenia. Myelography was non-diagnostic. A
presumptive diagnosis of lupus was made and she was
treated with pulsed methylprednisolone and
cyclophosphamide. In spite of treatment, her symptoms
continued to get worse.

Examination

There were no cutaneous stigmata of lupus. Cognitive assessment was normal.
Examination of the cranial nerves and upper limbs was also normal. The lower
abdominal reflexes were absent. In the lower limbs, tone was increased with
sustained clonus at both ankles. Power was normal. Reflexes were pathologically
brisk and both plantar responses were extensor. Vibration sense was absent to
the iliac crests but examination of the other sensory modalities was normal.

Investigations

MRI of the spinal cord showed evidence of intrinsic signal change between T6
and the conus. Graded echographic sequences also suggested a serpiginous
lesion on the cord surface. Subsequent spinal angiography with selective
injection of the intercostal arteries confirmed the presence of a dural

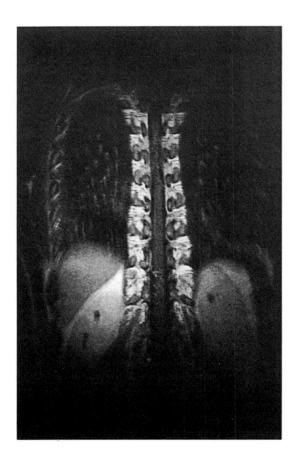

Figure 11 Spinal arteriovenous malformation. Characteristic serpiginous lesion on the cord surface demonstrated on an MRI scan.

arteriovenous shunt at the level of T12 on the right. The shunt was closely associated with the neural foramen and there was evidence of reflux into epidural and spinal veins. In view of these findings, the shunt was successfully embolised by selective catheterisation of the T12 intercostal artery. Subsequent to this procedure the venous phase of angiography was seen to normalise, indicating successful closure of the fistula.

Diagnosis	Spinal dural arteriovenous fistula and systemic lupus erythematosus

Commentary by Dr Wendy J Taylor

Spinal arteriovenous shunts draining via intrathecal veins were first described by Kendall and Logue in 1977. These durally based shunts are rare lesions, typically occurring in elderly men, presenting after protracted investigation for either spinal canal stenosis or intermittent claudication. Usually the progressive nature of the symptoms and late presentation result in only partially reversible ischaemic cord damage. Investigations include magnetic resonance imaging, where abnormal vessels may be visualised along with high signal on the T2 weighted sequence in the conus medullaris (Figure 11). The definitive investigation is spinal angiography where demonstration of the abnormal shunt can be identified along with the typical appearances of delayed venous phase anatomy, when the anterior spinal axis is opacified with contrast medium. This particular patient was unusual in that her age and sex precipitated rapid investigation and discovery of the aetiology of her symptoms. The association of lupus with dural arteriovenous shunts is not recognised, but one of the putative reasons for the development of these dural shunts is thrombosis of the spinal radicular veins. Therefore the increased thrombotic tendency in this patient may have been of aetiological significance. Treatment is obliteration of the shunt either by surgical or endovascular means. Usually, we recommend anticoagulation following the procedure to prevent further thrombosis.

Reference

Kendall BL, Logue L. Spinal epidural angiomatous malformations draining into intrathecal veins. *Neuroradiology* 1977;**13**:181–9.

CASE 19

History	A 27-year-old woman presented with a 3-month history of worsening headaches. These were especially severe in the mornings and associated with nausea and vomiting. She also noticed an abrupt onset of deafness in the right ear with subsequent vertigo, unsteadiness and intermittent horizontal diplopia. She had previously been well and there was no family history of note.

Examination

Higher cortical functions were normal. Visual acuities were 6/18 (corrected) left and 6/6 (corrected) right. There was bilateral enlargement of the blind spots. Fundoscopy revealed gross swelling of the optic discs. Eye movements were full with sustained nystagmus on right lateral gaze. Fifth and seventh nerve function was normal. There was right-sided sensorineural deafness. Pharyngeal sensation was diminished on the right. The palate was deviated to the left. There was a dysphonic quality to her voice with a weak cough. Shoulder shrug and tongue movements were normal. There were no abnormal findings in the peripheral nervous system. Cerebellar function was normal, except that the patient found it difficult to perform tandem walking. Hallpike's manoeuvre was negative.

Investigations

A CT scan of the brain revealed a large hyperdense mass lying posterior to the right cerebellopontine angle. There was displacement of the brain stem with associated hydrocephalus. This lesion was confirmed on MRI. The images revealed a central core of low signal. There was associated secondary herniation of the cerebellar tonsils to C1. The internal auditory meatus was not expanded. The patient subsequently underwent ventricular shunting followed by a posterior fossa craniectomy and excision of the tumour. Histologically this had the appearance of a meningioma with increased mitotic figures, indicating a degree of malignancy.

> **Diagnosis**   Infratentorial meningioma

Commentary by Dr Peter Rudge

The vast majority of infratentorial meningiomas are seen in women and it is disappointing that such a high proportion still present after the lesion has become extremely large. The hearing loss in this patient is typical of a cerebellopontine (CP) angle tumour and the sudden onset is common, and perhaps indicative of a vascular aetiology. The initial hearing loss in these patients has a peripheral quality, although sensory neural features develop at a

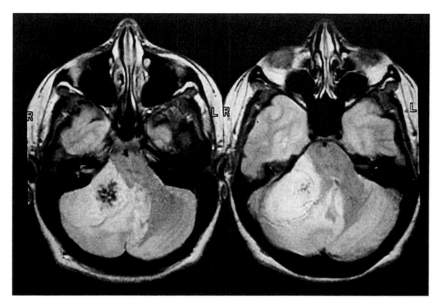

Figure 12 Infratentorial meningioma. T2 weighted MRI scan showing a central core of low signal in the right cerebello-pontine angle.

later stage. Meningiomas frequently cause much less hearing loss than acoustic schwannomas, presumably due to their anatomical location – the majority of meningiomas do not arise within the internal auditory meatus. A pointer to the true diagnosis in this case was the lower cranial nerve signs. Pharyngeal sensory loss due to ninth nerve involvement never occurs with VIII nerve schwannomas and vagal involvement is extremely rare. The nystagmus is of particular interest in that it was first degree to the right, the same side as the tumour. This indicates a large mass impinging upon the right side of the pons or the cerebellum. In contrast, an acoustic schwannoma characteristically causes a vestibular type nystagmus to the opposite side, evolving to an ipsilateral gaze-evoked nystagmus. Typically, CP angle tumours do not cause positional nystagmus. Sophisticated neuro-otological tests have, to some extent, been superseded by MRI (Figure 12). Nevertheless, the degree of vestibular malfunction, particularly on caloric testing, is much less in meningiomas than in acoustic schwannomas and the brainstem auditory evoked potentials are often surprisingly normal in these tumours, contrasting with their extreme sensitivity in acoustic schwannomas. The morbidity from operative intervention in these cases is still disappointingly high.

Reference

Robertson K, Rudge P. The differential diagnosis: cerebellopontine angle lesions. *J Neurol Sci* 1983;**60**:1–21.

CASE 20

History	A 47-year-old man developed a sharp pain over the left sternal edge exacerbated by coughing. The pain subsequently extended to the medial border of his left arm with associated numbness. He noticed that placing his left hand in hot water would induce an unpleasant dysasthaetic sensation. He had no other complaints. Seventeen years previously he had been involved in a road traffic accident with an associated whiplash injury and rib fractures.

Examination

The cranial nerves were normal. There were sparse fasciculations in the left deltoid muscle. There was weakness of the left upper limb. The left biceps and supinator jerks were absent. The rest of the examination was normal, apart from reduced temperature and pinprick sensation affecting the C4 to T6 dermatomes on the left.

Investigations

MRI examination of the spinal cord revealed a large syrinx extending from C3 to T10 to the left of the midline. There was no evidence of pathological enhancement with gadolinium and no features suggestive of an associated tumour.

Diagnosis	Syringomyelia

Commentary by Dr Christopher J Earl

The diagnosis of syringomyelia is one that used to be made on clinical grounds alone, perhaps with supporting but not definitive evidence from myelography, until the introduction of magnetic resonance imaging (MRI). Now, modern imaging techniques can demonstrate the spinal cord and the cavity within it and lead to a firm diagnosis (Figure 13).

In this case the MRI scan demonstrates not only the cavity and its situation but also enhancement with gadolinium showed nothing to suggest that the development of the cavity was due to the presence of an intramedullary tumour

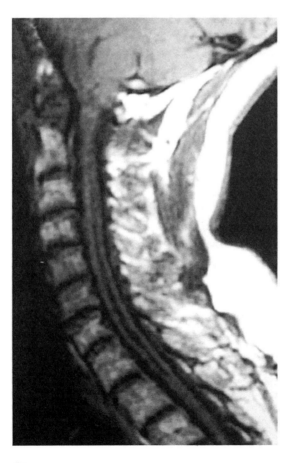

Figure 13 Syrinx. T1 weighted MRI scan demonstrating an extensive cavity within the cord.

in the spinal cord; such secondary cavitation does sometimes occur. In addition, there was no evidence of an Arnold–Chiari malformation, which is present in the majority of cases of idiopathic syringomyelia and may play a role in the pathogenesis of the cavity (Figure 14).

In the patient's history, the possible significance of the 'whiplash injury' must be considered. The development of cavities within the spinal cord following injury is well recognised. However, the injury is usually of sufficient severity to leave evidence of residual spinal cord damage, which was not the case here. With the benefit of hindsight, we can see that the first significant symptom was the pain on coughing felt over the anterior part of the left chest wall, later

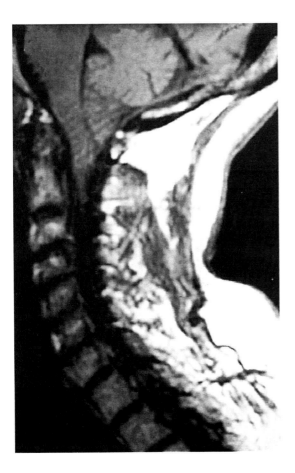

Figure 14
Arnold–Chiari malformation (Type 1). Saggital T1 weighted image showing inferior displacement of the cerebellar tonsils.

extending to the left upper limb. Pain on coughing and straining is a well recognised symptom in syringomyelia and is presumably related to a sharp rise in intracranial pressure transmitted to the cavity. A sudden deterioration of the physical signs may occur in similar circumstances. The signs in this case are all consistent with an intramedullary cord lesion involving the grey matter of the cervical cord. Occasional fasciculations over the deltoid indicate some involvement of the anterior horn cells, a common feature of this condition. Absence of reflexes is the result of grey matter involvement at the base of the posterior horn and may be the earliest sign of a developing syrinx. The impairment of pain and temperature sensation over the C4 to T6 dermatomes on the left is also consistent with involvement of cells at the base of the left posterior horn from which arise secondary neurones that cross the midline and ascend in the spinothalamic tract on the right side of the spinal cord.

Reference

Williams, B. On the pathogenesis of syringomyelia: a review. *J Roy Soc Med* 1980;**73**:798–806.

CASE 21

History	A 55-year-old Asian man was admitted to hospital with a 24-hour history of lethargy, confusion, agitation and headache. His alcohol consumption was excessive and his family confirmed that his average daily intake was over 10 units. He had developed non-insulin-dependent diabetes 6 years earlier. Following admission to hospital he developed generalised tonic–clonic seizures followed by a right hemiplegia.

Examination

The patient was agitated and confused. He had marked neck stiffness and was pyrexial (39°C). There was no evidence of a rash or other stigmata of a vasculitis or chronic liver disease. Neurological examination revealed a right hemiplegia with an associated right extensor plantar response.

Investigations

Investigation results are summarised in Table 2. Gram stain showed Gram-positive bacillae, subsequently confirmed to be *Listeria* on blood culture. A CT scan showed evidence of an infarct in left middle cerebral artery territory.

Diagnosis	*Listeria* meningitis complicated by stroke

Commentary by Dr Nicholas A Losseff

Alcohol may affect the nervous system in many ways and any alcoholic attending the Emergency Department should not be assumed only to be intoxicated. Of

Table 2 Haematological and biochemical investigations	
haemoglobin	9.8 g/dl
MCV	104 fl
ESR	104 mm/h
platelets	632 × 10⁹/l
neutrophils	11.4 × 10⁹/l
ALP	201 IU/l
ALT	69 IU/l
γGT	223 IU/l
CRP	106 mg/l
CSF protein	2 g/l
CSF white cell count	150 (60% polymorphs:40% lymphocytes)
CSF glucose	7 mmol/l
plasma glucose	18 mmol/l

particular importance is Wernicke's encephalopathy, which must be considered in any individual with unexplained confusion or a depressed level of consciousness, particularly in the presence of eye signs; early treatment with high-dose thiamine is mandatory. Wernicke's encephalopathy is unlikely in this patient with fever and neck stiffness and the clinical differential diagnosis is broad including tumour, abscess, subdural haematoma, encephalitis, meningitis and hyperosmolar diabetic coma, all of which may present with focal neurological signs. It is clear from the clinical features that this was not a simple cerebrovascular accident as the lethargy, confusion and agitation preceded the right hemiparesis. Although pyrexia commonly accompanies stroke, neck stiffness is rare unless there is also subarachnoid blood or brain herniation is imminent. Hence lumbar puncture was essential here and it revealed the diagnosis of bacterial meningitis. If Gram-positive bacilli had not been demonstrated, it would have been essential to consider TB in view of the patient's ethnic origin. CNS listeriosis takes two main forms and predominantly, but not exclusively, affects the immunocompromised. This patient is at risk

68

because of excess alcohol consumption and diabetes. At one end of the spectrum *Listeria* cause a meningitic illness usually with a markedly abnormal CSF. At the other end, a brainstem encephalitis occurs with cranial nerve palsies and long tract signs secondary to listerial micro-abscesses. In this form, the CSF can be quite indolent. In all cases stroke may be a complicating factor. Treatment is with high-dose ampicillin with or without gentamicin.

Reference

John JF. Listeria monocytogenes. In: Vinken PJ, Bruyn GW, Klawans HL, Eds. *Handbook of Clinical Neurology 8 (52) Microbial Disease.* New York: Elsevier Science; 1988:89–101.

CASE 22

History	A 37-year-old man was noted to have delayed speech in infancy. At the age of 5 years bilateral sensorineural deafness was noted on routine screening. He was otherwise well until the age of 13 years when he developed transient attacks of dysphasia followed by a throbbing headache. Eight years later he developed generalised tonic–clonic seizures and a progressive gait ataxia. He had also noticed jerking of all four limbs without impairment of consciousness. At the age of 31 years his speech became dysarthric and his coordination deteriorated markedly. His seizures and jerks were felt to be photosensitive. His mother and three siblings were affected by a similar illness.

Examination

The patient was of short stature but there were no other dysmorphic features. Cranial nerve examination revealed normal eye movements and no fundal or pupillary abnormalities. He had mild bilateral lower motor neurone facial weakness, sensorineural deafness and dysarthria. There was marked weakness of neck flexion. Examination of the peripheral nervous system revealed proximal wasting and frequent myoclonic jerks with stimulus sensitivity. There was proximal upper and lower limb weakness and arreflexia. Plantar responses were flexor. He had a stocking distribution loss of temperature and pinprick sensation affecting both lower limbs. Testing of cerebellar function was difficult due to frequent myoclonic jerks but there was evidence of additional upper and lower limb ataxia.

Investigations

Full blood count, ESR, urea and electrolytes, liver function tests and thyroid function tests were normal. Random lactate level was 4.42 mmol/l (normal range 0.5–1.65 mmol/l), pyruvate level was 98 μmol/l (normal), and the lactate:pyruvate ratio was 45 (normal range 10–20). EEG investigation showed moderately severe abnormalities of background rhythm with bilateral following photic responses. Evoked potential recording demonstrated the presence of giant SSEPs. Nerve conduction studies suggested the presence of an axonal sensory neuropathy with reduced amplitude sensory nerve action potentials and normal conduction velocities. EMG recordings were characterised by increased insertional activity with some large polyphasic units on recruitment. A muscle biopsy showed ragged red fibres and cytochrome C oxidase negative fibres consistent with a defect of mitochondrial DNA (mtDNA). Mitochondrial DNA analysis confirmed the presence of the 8344 mutation in muscle and blood.

Diagnosis   Myoclonus epilepsy with ragged red fibres (MERRF)

Commentary by Dr Michael G Hanna

At the age of 37 years this patient has a combination of myoclonus, cerebellar ataxia and epilepsy and therefore falls within the syndrome known as progressive myoclonic ataxia with epilepsy (PMA/E). The differential diagnosis is potentially wide but five disorders in particular should be considered. These are: Unverricht–Lundborg disease, Lafora body disease, sialidosis, neuronal ceroid lipofucinosis and myoclonus epilepsy with ragged red fibres (MERRF). The slowly progressive natural history, the deafness, and the clinical signs of myopathy and neuropathy all suggest that MERRF is the likely diagnosis. MERRF is one of the recognised mitochondrial disease phenotypes and is due to impaired mitochondrial respiratory chain function. The constant clinical features in its fully developed form are progressive myoclonus which is cortical in origin, cerebellar ataxia, generalised seizures and myopathy. The myoclonus and ataxia are usually the dominant clinical features while the seizures and myopathy tend to be less prominent. Additional features, some of which this patient had, may include short stature, optic atrophy, sensorineural deafness, dementia, hemicranial headache, pyramidal signs and a sensory neuropathy. Some cases of MERRF have stroke-like episodes suggesting an overlap with another recognised mitochondrial disease phenotype known as MELAS (mitochondrial encephalomyopathy, lactic

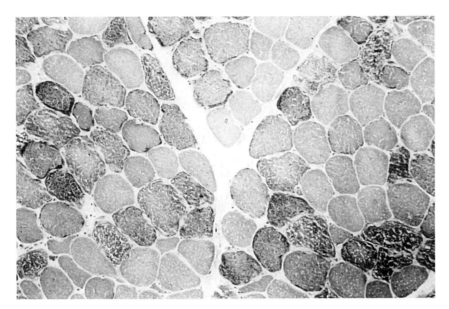

Figure 15 *MERRF. Gomori trichrome stain of muscle section showing abundant red staining of 'ragged red' fibres. Courtesy of Dr M G Hanna.*

acidosis and stroke-like episodes). MERRF is maternally inherited but the severity of the disease may vary considerably in different relatives ranging from deafness alone to the full-blown MERRF syndrome. Most cases of MERRF have been shown to be associated with a point mutation in a mitochondrial transfer RNA lysine gene at position 8344 in mitochondrial DNA. The elevated lactate and lactate:pyruvate ratio indicate impaired respiratory chain function and the evoked potentials confirm the cortical origin of the myoclonus. The most useful investigations are mitochondrial DNA analysis and muscle biopsy. The 8344 mutation is usually detectable in blood as well as muscle. This is in contrast to some other mitochondrial DNA mutations such as the common MELAS mutation at position 3243 which is more reliably detected in muscle. The muscle biopsy findings in this case are typical with ragged red fibres, which represent areas of focal mitochondrial proliferation, and fibres with absent cytochrome c oxidase staining (Figure 15). Currently there is no effective therapy and treatment is supportive.

Reference

Seibel P, Deogoul F, Bonne G, *et al*. Genetic, biochemical and pathophysiological characterisation of a familial mitochondrial encephalomyopathy (MERRF). *J Neurol Sci* 1991;**105**:217–24.

CASE 23

History A 42-year-old man was a known intravenous drug abuser. Ten years previously he had asked for an HIV test and this was positive. He had been completely well until 2 years previously when he noticed an abnormal sensation affecting the right side of his body including the face. Twelve months later he noticed a progressive gait disturbance secondary to right lower limb weakness. This was followed by the insidious development of a language disorder characterised by word finding difficulties. He had received an 8-week course of anti-toxoplasmosis treatment without benefit.

Examination

The patient looked well and was apyrexial. There was evidence of oral and pharyngeal candidiasis. His speech was non-fluent with relative preservation of comprehension. He had difficulty in repeating words and phrases. There was clear evidence of dyslexia and dyscalculia but no dysgraphia or finger agnosia. Cranial nerve examination was normal apart from reduced light touch and pinprick sensation over the right side of the face. Tone was increased in the right sided limbs with concomitant mild pyramidal weakness and reflex asymmetry. Both plantar responses were flexor. Sensory testing revealed diminished sensation to all modalities on the right. There was no evidence of limb apraxia and there were no cerebellar signs.

Investigations

An MRI scan of the brain showed an area of abnormal mixed signal in the left frontoparietal area extending from the cortex to the deep white matter. There was extensive surrounding vasogenic oedema. A second lesion was noted anterior to the left frontal horn. Results of the full blood count are shown in Table 3.

Table 3 Haematological investigations	
haemoglobin	9.5 g/dl
ESR	99 mm/h
lymphocytes	$1.0 \times 10^9/l$
neutrophils	$1.8 \times 10^9/l$
CD4 count	$0.04 \times 10^9/l$
CD4:CD8 ratio	0.05 (normal range 0.38–3.39)

Toxoplasma, histoplasmosis, syphilis and cysticercosis serology were negative. Polymerase chain reaction for *Toxoplasmosis gondii* was negative. Immunoglobulins were normal. A stereotactic biopsy of the larger lesion was performed and this showed clear histological evidence of a cerebral B cell lymphoma.

Diagnosis   Cerebral lymphoma associated with HIV

Commentary by Professor Michael J G Harrison

Cerebral lymphomas are difficult to distinguish from toxoplasma abscesses in patients with AIDS (Figure 16). Both may present with the subacute development of focal neurological deficits with or without the effects of raised intracranial pressure. Both can produce multiple ring-enhancing mass lesions on CT or MRI. Extension of the mass along the ventricular wall is highly suggestive of lymphoma when present (Figure 17). Thallium scans may also help in discrimination as a very high uptake of tracer is usually found to relate to lymphoma. Toxoplasma serological tests are not decisive. The lymphoma is related to Epstein–Barr virus (EBV) infection and detection of EBV by the polymerase chain reaction (PCR) in the CSF is a valuable diagnostic pointer. However, it is often not safe to lumbar puncture these patients with mass lesions. Therefore it is often necessary to consider a brain biopsy if there is

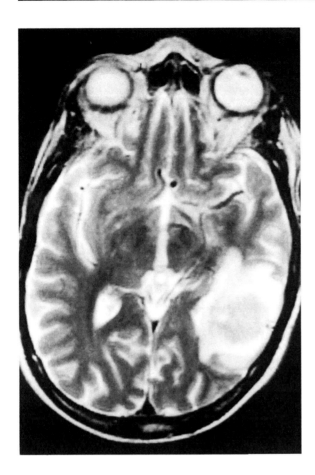

Figure 16 *Cerebral lymphoma. T2 weighted MRI scan demonstrating solid mass lesion with surrounding high density change secondary to oedema. Courtesy of Professor MJG Harrison.*

neither clinical or radiological response to anti-toxoplasma treatment over 2 to 3 weeks. Radiotherapy can reverse neurological deficits in lymphoma and is worth considering if the patient's general condition is good. Unfortunately, the overall prognosis is poor as patients with cerebral lymphoma often have very low CD4 counts, as in our case, and usually succumb to opportunistic infections and general debility within three to four months.

77

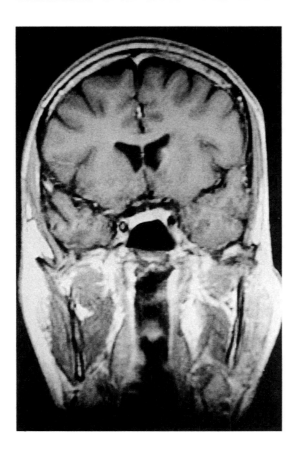

Figure 17 Cerebral lymphoma. T1 weighted image showing a small nodule spreading along the ventricular wall. Courtesy of Professor MJG Harrison.

Reference

Miller RF, *et al*. Comparison of Magnetic Resonance Imaging, Thallium-201 SPECT Scanning and Laboratory Analyses for Diagnosis of Focal CNS Lesions in AIDS. *J Neurol Neurosurg Psychiatry* 1998 (In press).

CASE 24

History   A 54-year-old man was admitted to hospital with a 3-month history of reduced exercise tolerance with particular difficulty climbing stairs. In addition, he complained of exertional dyspnoea and 4-pillow orthopnoea. He had no dysphagia or dysarthria. A chest X-ray suggested collapse and consolidation at both lung bases with bilateral elevation of the diaphragm. He developed type II respiratory failure and was therefore intubated and ventilated. He was treated with antibiotics and physiotherapy but in spite of this it was impossible to wean him from the ventilator. His past medical and family history were unremarkable. He was a non-smoker and had continued working as a carpenter until 3 weeks before his admission.

Examination

The patient had a hyperlordotic gait and a positive Trendelenburg's test. Cranial nerve examination was normal apart from weakness of orbicularis oris. There was no tongue fasciculation or wasting and the neck flexor muscles were of normal power. He had upper and lower limb proximal wasting and weakness with scapular winging. There were no fasciculations and reflexes were normal in the upper and lower limbs. Both plantar responses were flexor and sensory examination was unremarkable. Vital capacity was 1.1 litre erect falling to 500 ml supine. Paradoxical breathing was present.

Investigations

Creatine kinase levels were normal. Routine haematology, biochemistry and thyroid function were normal. EMG showed myopathic changes with superimposed polyphasic units compatible with denervation. Vacuolated lymphocytes were seen on a peripheral blood film (Figure 18). A muscle biopsy

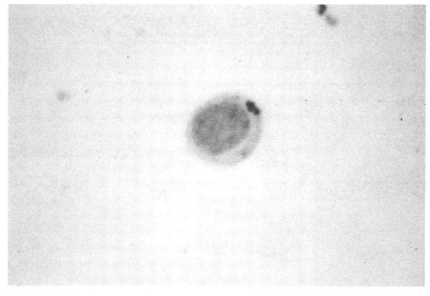

Figure 18 *Acid maltase deficiency. Vacuolated lymphocyte. Courtesy of Dr JM Land.*

demonstrated vacuolation in some fibres with positive staining for glycogen and acid phosphatase.

Diagnosis   Acid maltase deficiency

Commentary by Dr John A Morgan-Hughes

Acid maltase deficiency (glycogen storage disease type II) is inherited as an autosomal recessive trait with three clinically distinct variants. The fatal infantile form (Pompe's disease) presents soon after birth with severe hypotonic weakness, variable enlargement of the liver and tongue and massive cardiomegaly. It is rapidly progressive and leads to death from cardiorespiratory failure in the first or second year. The childhood variant is largely restricted to skeletal muscle. Motor milestones may be delayed owing to weakness of the limb girdle muscles and trunk. There may be calf hypertrophy and nasal speech due to palatal weakness. Involvement of the respiratory muscles and diaphragm is common and eventually leads to death from respiratory insufficiency in the second or third decades. The adult variant begins between the second and fifth decades with slowly progressive weakness of the limb girdle muscles and trunk. Chronic ventilatory insufficiency due to diaphragmatic weakness is an early manifestation in one-third of cases. It can be detected by measuring the vital capacity in the upright and supine positions or by recording transdiaphragmatic pressures. The differential diagnosis includes limb girdle muscular dystrophy, polymyositis, late onset nemaline myopathy and motor neurone disease. The serum creatine kinase level may be moderately elevated. The EMG is myopathic and vacuolar glycogen storage is present in blood lymphocytes. Muscle biopsy shows scattered fibres containing multiple vacuoles which are packed with glycogen and stain intensely for the lysosomal marker enzyme acid phosphatase. Acid maltase activity in lymphocytes and muscle is often undetectable in the fatal infantile form but in adult onset cases there is usually some residual activity. Acid maltase (acid α-glucosidase) is a lysosomal enzyme which hydrolyses the α-1,4 and the α-1,6 linkages of glycogen, maltose and linear oligosaccharides yielding glucose. It is expressed in all tissues and is encoded by a single gene which has been mapped to chromosome 17q23. The protein is synthesised as a precursor with an N-terminal signal peptide and undergoes complex co-translational and post-translational processing in the endoplasmic reticulum and the Golgi with maturation in the primary lysosomes. DNA analysis in acid maltase deficiency has identified extensive genetic heterogeneity with small deletions, insertions, missense/nonsense mutations and splice site defects scattered throughout the coding sequence. Most adult cases are compound heterozygotes.

Reference

Wokke JH, Ausems MG, van der Boogard MJ. Genotype-phenotype correlation in adult onset acid maltase deficiency. *Ann Neurol* 1995;**38**:450–4.

CASE 25

History	A 32-year-old man had sustained his first generalised tonic clonic seizure 12 months previously. During recovery he was noted to be extremely aggressive and had to be restrained with handcuffs. He was taken to hospital and found to be pyrexial. He was treated with intravenous acyclovir and a lumbar puncture was performed, which was normal. Three months later he began to bite his tongue voluntarily without impairment of consciousness. Some of these tongue lacerations required suturing. As a consequence, he found eating rather painful and began to lose weight. Following this, he developed orolingual choreiform movements. His work performance had declined over the previous 12 months but he was otherwise well. There was no family history of neurological disease. He had never been prescribed neuroleptics.

Examination

General examination was normal. The patient had widespread choreiform movements with additional orolingual dystonia. His eye movements and fundal examination were normal. The rest of the neurological examination was unremarkable.

Investigations

Routine haematology, biochemistry and thyroid function were normal. The creatine kinase level was 735 IU/l (normal range 20–200 IU/l). Uric acid level was normal. A wet blood film demonstrated 9% acanthocytes. Vitamin E levels, cholesterol and triglyceride levels were normal. Lipid electrophoresis was normal. An MRI scan of the brain was normal. Neuropsychometric testing was compatible with a degree of generalised cognitive decline. Nerve conduction studies and EMG were normal. EEG examination showed diffuse slow wave activity but no epileptiform discharges.

Diagnosis Neuroacanthocytosis

Commentary by Dr Andrew J Lees

Neuroacanthocytosis presents most commonly in the fourth decade of life, classically with stereotyped orofacial dyskinesias associated with tongue, lip and cheek biting. Vocalisations, personality change, a mild axonal neuropathy with arreflexia and generalised chorea or dystonia are also frequent. A seizure is a common presenting feature (one-third of all cases have epilepsy); half of the patients have cognitive blunting and a few develop a late parkinsonian syndrome. The diagnosis may be missed, even when it is considered in the differential because of a failure to examine at least three fresh blood films; films reported as showing crenation or anisopoikilocytosis should be deemed suspicious. In doubtful cases, phase contrast microscopy or scanning electron microscopy may be useful in distinguishing acanthocytes from echinocytes. In the appropriate clinical context, ≥3% acanthocytes is significant. Almost all patients have a moderately elevated creatine kinase level. The genetics are unclear; both autosomal recessive and dominant inheritance are considered and there appears to be a 2:1 male preponderance. One family has been described with the McLeod phenotype. This condition is caused by a mutant gene on the short arm of the X chromosome, and is associated with abnormal Kell blood antigens, acanthocytosis and subclinical myopathy. Treatment of the dyskinesias and seizures is very difficult and slow but relentless progression of disability is the norm.

Reference

Hardie RJ, Pullon HW, Harding AE, *et al*. Neuroacanthocytosis: a clinical, haematological and pathological study of 19 cases. *Brain* 1991;**114**:13–49.

CASE 26

History   A 30-year-old pianoforte maker was admitted to the
National Hospital in 1923. Three months previously he had
developed a gradual onset of weakness affecting his right
sided limbs. He attended the medical baths at Southend and
experienced a temporary improvement in his symptoms but
following this he deteriorated and became bed-bound. He
also noticed some transient shaking affecting his right side
which subsided after two weeks. His past medical history
was unremarkable and there was no relevant family history.
He was a smoker but did not abuse alcohol. Examination at
that time revealed a fit looking man who had good colour
and was clean shaven. His gums were in good condition and
his teeth, although slightly decayed and stained, were all his
own. He was 'quite intelligent' and answered questions well.
Neurological abnormalities were confined to the limbs. His
right arm had a spastic increase in tone and brisk reflexes
but no weakness. In the lower limbs he had a pyramidal
increase in tone (worse on the right than on the left) with a
pyramidal pattern of weakness in the right lower limb. There
was clear reflex asymmetry (brisker on the right than on the
left) with bilaterally extensor plantar responses. There were
no definite sensory abnormalities. His gait was abnormal
with marked stiffness of the right leg and his foot was noted
to scrape the floor. He spent 48 days in hospital and during
the admission had a lumbar puncture. This showed clear and
colourless fluid with 10 cells and a total protein of 0.015%.
The Wassermann reaction and Lange test were negative. The
patient improved after discharge but was unable to walk
unassisted for a further 2 years. He was readmitted 40 years
later having been well until 18 months previously. From that
time he noticed a progressive weakness of his right lower
limb and loss of dexterity of the right hand.

Examination

The patient had evidence of mild global cognitive impairment. The cranial nerves were normal. He had a moderately severe pyramidal weakness affecting his right arm and both legs. His right plantar response was extensor, the left was equivocal. He was unable to walk.

PROGRESS

His condition deteriorated over the next 2 years in a progressive fashion. He developed a severe quadriparesis and became bed-bound. He died 3 years later from bronchopneumonia.

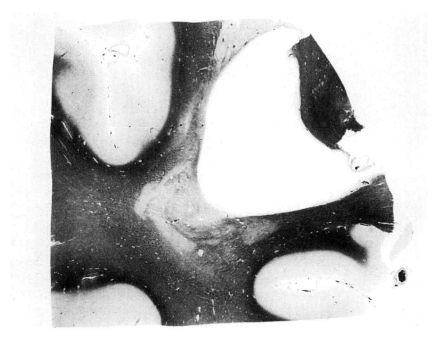

Figure 19 Multiple sclerosis. Coronal section through part of the lateral ventricle and adjacent white matter. The distribution of the areas of myelin pallor are characteristic of multiple sclerosis. Courtesy of Professor WI McDonald.

POSTMORTEM FINDINGS

The spinal cord was normal. The lateral and third ventricles were enlarged, with marked thinning of the corpus callosum. White matter abnormalities were noted throughout the subcortical regions with relative sparing of the brain stem. Histological sections from these regions showed a widespread loss of myelinated nerve fibres and local swelling of the myelin sheaths (Figure 19). The blood vessels were normal.

Diagnosis   Multiple sclerosis

Commentary by Professor W Ian McDonald

In this patient the distribution of lesions at post mortem was characteristic of multiple sclerosis and the histological changes were compatible with a quiescent phase of the disease. Axonal loss, which may be extensive, is common late in the course of multiple sclerosis and plays an important part in determining the irrecoverable deficit. A diagnosis of disseminated (multiple) sclerosis was made at presentation, although this would not be possible now: modern criteria require that there must have been at least two episodes of neurological disturbance of the kind seen in multiple sclerosis and evidence of neurological abnormalities attributable to white matter damage at not less than two necessarily separate sites in the central nervous system. The original finding of ten cells/mm^3 in the CSF is common in multiple sclerosis. The Lange test (which depends on alterations in the CSF immunoglobulin G, now recognised as oligoclonal bands at electrophoresis) was negative and so gave no additional diagnostic support. The interval of some 38 years between the first episode and the onset of the secondary progressive phase of the illness is exceptionally long and serves to illustrate the enormous variability in the course of multiple sclerosis, the difficulty in predicting the future after a single episode of neurological disturbance, and the necessity of large-scale double-blind controlled trials in assessing treatment.

Reference

Compston DAS, Ed. *McAlpines multiple sclerosis,* 3rd edn. London: WB Saunders and Co; 1998.

CASE 27

History   A 66-year-old woman had presented with painless transient visual loss affecting the right eye which lasted for 20 minutes and resolved without sequelae. Two years later she inadvertently covered her left eye and noticed diminished visual acuity on the right with impairment of colour vision. The acuity in her right eye progressively deteriorated over the next 18 months to perception of light only on the affected side. There was no associated pain. She also had rheumatoid arthritis and had been treated with gold and steroids in the past but no other disease modifying agents had been used. Her family history was unremarkable. She had no unusual dietary habits and did not consume alcohol to excess.

Examination

The patient had a 2 mm proptosis of the right eye. The right pupil was larger than the left and there was a right relative afferent pupillary defect. Fundoscopy revealed optic atrophy on the right with two retinal choroidal collateral vessels. Visual acuity was perception of light on the right; 6/6, N5 on the left. There was no obvious field loss and the rest of the neurological examination was normal.

Investigations

Routine haematology, biochemistry and thyroid function were normal. The ESR was 56 mm/hour. Rheumatoid factor was positive in high titre. An MRI scan of the brain and orbits demonstrated an enlarged right optic nerve with high signal extending from the intraorbital portion as far as the chiasm. The lesion was noted to be partially cystic within the chiasm (Figure 20). There was also pathological gadolinium enhancement of the lesion confined to the optic chiasm.

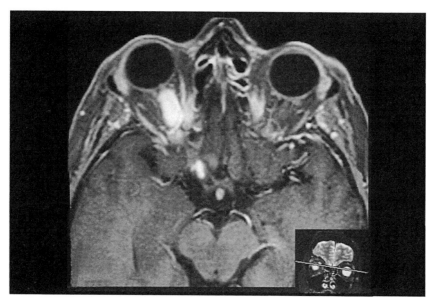

Figure 20 *Optic nerve glioma. T1 weighted enhanced MRI scan showing enlarged right optic nerve with signal change extending to the optic chiasm.*

The patient subsequently underwent a right transorbital optic nerve biopsy. This was characterised by atypical nuclei within the optic nerve and increased cellularity consistent with a low grade glioma.

Diagnosis   Primary optic nerve glioma

Commentary by Professor W Ian McDonald

Primary optic nerve glioma is a rare tumour, which almost always presents in childhood. Histologically, it is a low-grade astrocytoma which may extend intracranially into the chiasm without giving outward signs that it has done so. The commonest presentation is with visual loss (or its consequence, such as squint in young children) and proptosis. Examination reveals optic atrophy and occasionally tumour at the optic nerve head. Cilioretinal vessels may be seen, indicating that the lesion is of long standing. When the hypothalamus is involved in childhood, precocious puberty may occur. Neurofibromatosis is associated in approximately 50% of cases. High resolution MRI of the optic nerve and chiasmal region is the investigation of choice. The childhood cases fall into two groups: one in which the condition changes little or not at all over many years, the other in which it progresses over a matter of months. These patterns determine management. After clinical diagnosis, patients should be reassessed three or four times in the first year. If the condition is stationary the follow-up intervals can be lengthened gradually and conservative management continued. If progression is rapid, excision biopsy of the optic nerve should be performed once useful vision is lost in that eye. The role of chemotherapy and radiotherapy have not been defined. The latter appears to have slowed progression in some but not all cases. Treatment is not indicated unless there is clear evidence of progression.

Reference

Wright JE, McNab AA, McDonald WI. Optic nerve glioma and the management of optic nerve tumours in the young. *Br J Ophthalmol* 1989;**73**:967–74.

CASE 28

History　A 78-year-old woman gave a 15-year history of unsteadiness on standing. She had never fallen but found that she had to lean on objects to maintain her balance. She had also noticed the development of a postural upper limb tremor which disappeared on lying down or sitting. There was no past medical or family history of neurological illness.

Examination

When the patient stood up she swayed markedly and demonstrated frequent postural adjustments of her toes. Her gait was normal but she was unable to tandem walk slowly, although this did improve at pace. On standing she developed a postural tremor of the outstretched upper limbs with an additional tremor visible at the patellae. On auscultation over the knees with a stethoscope, a characteristic thumping sound was heard. There were no extrapyramidal or cerebellar abnormalities.

Investigations

EMG recordings taken when the patient was standing demonstrated a synchronous 14 Hz tremor in upper and lower limbs which disappeared when the patient was lifted off the floor.

Diagnosis　Primary orthostatic tremor

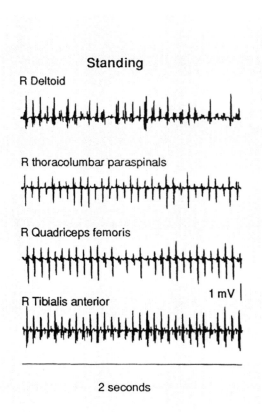

Standing

R Deltoid

R thoracolumbar paraspinals

R Quadriceps femoris

1 mV

R Tibialis anterior

2 seconds

Figure 21 Primary orthostatic tremor. Typical surface EMG demonstrating a synchronous 16 Hz tremor in all muscle groups.

Commentary by Dr Peter Brown

Primary orthostatic tremor was first described by Heilman in 1984. The tremor appears in muscles utilised in postural tasks (e.g. the leg muscles on standing) and has a high frequency of around 14 to 16 Hz (Figure 21). Balance is therefore compromised by a partially fused contraction of postural muscles, resulting in a feeling of instability and an intolerance of standing still. The abnormalities on examination are subtle and are often overlooked, leading to a diagnosis of a functional balance disorder. On standing still, some patients exhibit a fine fast tremor in the lower limbs, most evident around the superior aspect of the patellae. The diagnosis is simply confirmed by auscultation with the diaphragm of a stethoscope over the muscles of the lower limbs. A characteristic regular fast thumping sound is heard, rather like that of a distant helicopter. Importantly, the tremor disappears when muscles are no longer posturally active, such as when a standing patient is lifted off the floor or when the patient walks at a pace. The condition is occasionally seen with an additional upper limb tremor. It is important to distinguish primary orthostatic tremor from Parkinson's disease which may also present with an isolated leg tremor, although here this is usually at rest, asymmetric and at a much lower frequency. The cause of primary orthostatic tremor is unknown. Some authors have suggested that it may represent a variant of essential tremor. The response to drug treatment is generally disappointing, although clonazepam and levodopa are occasionally helpful. The prognosis is good, with the vast majority of patients remaining ambulant.

Reference

Britton TC, Thompson PD, van der Kamp, *et al*. Primary orthostatic tremor: Further observations in 6 cases. *J Neurol* 1992;**239**:209–17.

CASE 29

History	A 67-year-old man developed a flu-like illness with anorexia and weight loss. He also described a right temporal/parietal headache with minimal scalp tenderness. On the day of admission he developed sudden painless visual loss affecting the right eye. He described this as 'like a curtain coming down over his visual field'. Examination at that stage revealed diminished visual acuity on the right (hand movements), 6/9 (corrected) on the left. The right optic disc was swollen with a right relative afferent pupillary defect. He was started on treatment with intravenous steroids but 2 days later complained of two episodes of transient visual loss affecting the left eye, followed 24 hours later by permanent painless visual loss.

Examination

Light reactions were absent in both pupils. Visual acuities were hand movements in the right eye, no perception of light in the left. There was an inferior altitudinal field defect on the right. The right optic disc was swollen. The left disc was normal but there was retinal pallor. There was no temporal artery tenderness and the rest of the examination was normal.

Investigations

Routine haematology and biochemistry were normal. The ESR was 83 mm/hour. Temporal artery biopsy showed evidence of luminal occlusion with intimal degeneration. There was a marked inflammatory infiltrate in the media with focal necrosis.

> **Diagnosis**   Giant cell arteritis with right anterior ischaemic optic
> neuropathy and left central retinal artery occlusion

Commentary by Dr Gordon T Plant

The initial presentation of this patient was classical of giant cell arteritis
presenting with loss of vision. Systemic symptoms including anorexia preceded
the development of acute unilateral visual loss, which was caused by an anterior
ischaemic optic neuropathy giving rise to acute swelling of the optic disc on that
side acutely. The diagnosis was confirmed on temporal artery biopsy by which
time appropriate treatment had been initiated. The subsequent progress is
remarkable for loss of vision in the other eye, despite this treatment.
Unfortunately, this is not uncommon in giant cell arteritis. I have observed
pulsation return in occluded superficial temporal arteries over about 1 week;
presumably the vessel in this case was on the point of occluding before
treatment was started. In my experience, the longest period between initiating
treatment and loss of vision in the other eye is 10 days. There is often some
evidence that the other eye is involved, for example transient obscurations of
vision on standing or the presence of cotton wool spots in the retina. The
second, more unusual feature is the fact that visual loss in the second eye was
due to an occlusion of the central retinal artery, rather than an anterior
ischaemic optic neuropathy. Involvement of the retinal and choroidal
circulations in giant cell arteritis is extremely common (in non-arteritic anterior
ischaemic optic neuropathy this does not occur) because the pathology extends
as far proximal as the ophthalmic artery itself and also involves the collateral
supply to the eye from branches of the external carotid artery. Usually, however,
there is ischaemic disc swelling and the visual loss is predominantly due to a
severe anterior ischaemic optic neuropathy.

Reference

Matzkin DC, Slamovits TL, Sachs R, Burde RM. Visual recovery in two patients after
intravenous methylprednisolone treatment of central retinal artery occlusion secondary
to giant cell arteritis. *Ophthalmol* 1992;**99**:68–71.

CASE 30

<table>
<tr>
<td>History</td>
<td>A 39-year-old woman presented with a 2-year history of predominantly sensory disturbance. After delivery of her first child she developed a burning sensation in her left foot with associated weakness. This resolved after 2 months but recurred 6 months later. In addition, she developed similar sensory symptoms in her right hand with loss of dexterity. She felt systemically unwell and lost 2 stones in weight over a 4-month period. She also complained of generalised joint pains and night sweats. Her past medical history was unremarkable, apart from the development of asthma at the age of 34. This had required one hospital admission and had responded to systemic steroid treatment.</td>
</tr>
</table>

Examination

There was no evidence of a vasculitis or arthropathy. Auscultation of the chest revealed a prominent expiratory wheeze. Neurological abnormalities were confined to the peripheral nervous system. There was no wasting or fasciculations. Both deltoid muscles were weak (grade 4) with additional weakness of the right finger abductors (grade 4). In the lower limbs, both hip flexors were weak (grade 4) and plantar flexion of the left foot was also abnormal (grade 3). Reflexes were present and plantar responses were flexor. Sensory examination was abnormal with loss of light touch, pinprick and temperature sensation over the dorsum of the left foot. There was no evidence of nerve hypertrophy.

Investigations

The results of the haematological investigations are shown in Table 4. Routine biochemistry and creatine kinase levels were normal. Urinalysis showed no casts or proteinuria. ANF and ANCA were negative. Rheumatoid factor titre was

Table 4 Haematological investigations	
haemoglobin	10.0 g/dl
ESR	96 mm/h
platelets	851 × 10⁹/l
eosinophils	15.5 × 10⁹/l (normal = 0–0.4 × 10⁹/l)

>20,480. The cryoglobulin test was negative and immunoglobulin levels were normal. The chest X-ray was normal. Nerve conduction studies revealed absent sensory action potentials affecting the right radial, left tibial and both sural nerves. The left posterior tibial compound muscle action potential was of low amplitude – 0.3 mV (5.5 mV on the right). Lower limb f-wave responses were normal. EMG showed chronic neurogenic changes in the left gastronemius. A nerve biopsy was not performed.

Diagnosis   Churg–Strauss syndrome causing mononeuritis multiplex

---

Commentary by Dr Hadi Manji

Although Churg–Strauss (CS) syndrome (allergic granulomatous angiitis) is the most likely diagnosis in a patient presenting with the triad of asthma, eosinophilia and a mononeuritis multiplex, this case has a number of unusual features. Clinically, pain was not a prominent symptom: this would be expected since the underlying pathophysiology in vasculitis is ischaemia. The reflexes were intact, although this could be explained by involvement of very distal or small nerve fibres. In 70% of patients with CS syndrome p-ANCA is positive and a high IgE level is to be expected, reflecting the underlying atopy – both of these were absent. The RhF was very high with no clinical evidence of rheumatoid arthritis (RhA), which is difficult to explain unless it was merely a non-specific marker of immunological stimulation. Vasculitic neuropathies in RhA usually

100

occur in the context of long-standing and severe joint disease. However, at least one case has been reported in the literature of peripheral nerve vasculitis, eosinophilia and high RhF titres, where the patient developed an inflammatory arthritis 5 years later. Raised RhF titres may be found in a variety of conditions including sarcoidosis, tuberculosis, sytemic lupus erythematosus and bacterial endocarditis. Particularly high levels may occur in Sjögren's syndrome and the macroglobulinaemias. Thus it would be useful to repeat the measurement and confirm the levels using one of the other methods of assay (latex fixation test, sheep agglutination test or ELISA). CS syndrome may be mimicked by parasitic infestations such as ascariasis and trichinosis with a vasculitis, eosinophilia and pulmonary symptoms. We are not given a travel history but it would be prudent to check the stools for ova and parasites and to perform the appropriate serological tests. Although a nerve biopsy was not performed in this case, it could have been recommended in view of the atypical features. Vasculitis is a histological diagnosis and for this reason a combined nerve and muscle biopsy is useful before embarking on long-term treatment with steroids or cyclophosphamide. CS usually responds well to corticosteroids.

Reference

Jennette JC, Falk RJ. Small vessel vasculitis. *N Engl J Med* 1997;**337**:1512–23.

CASE 31

History	A 49-year-old man presented with malaise, anaemia, weight loss and diarrhoea 10 years previously. A jejunal biopsy was performed at that stage and a diagnosis was reached. At the age of 47 he re-presented with a progressive history of hypersomnolence and impaired short-term memory. He also developed visual hallucinations. His cognitive problems worsened and he developed daily headaches with no features of raised intracranial pressure. He had previously been well and there was no family history of neurological disorders. His alcohol consumption was minimal.

Examination

General examination was normal with no skin rashes or arthropathy. His gait was ataxic. He had slowing of vertical saccadic eye movements and impaired convergence. Fundoscopy was normal. There were no lateralising signs or myoclonus and both plantar responses were flexor. Psychometric testing revealed marked deficits of frontal lobe function. There were no primitive reflexes.

Investigations

Routine haematology and biochemistry were normal. CSF analysis revealed a protein level of 1.79 g/l with 24 white cells (mononuclear), a normal glucose level and negative oligoclonal bands. Polymerase chain reaction was positive for tropheryma whippelii. An MRI scan of the brain showed generalised cerebral atrophy with a high signal lesion in the right olive which was non-enhancing.

Diagnosis	Whipple's disease

Commentary by Dr Adrian J Wills

In 1907 GH Whipple characterised an illness affecting mainly middle-aged Caucasian men. He described a clinical tetrad of weight loss, diarrhoea, arthralgia and abdominal pain. Subsequently, Black-Schaffer demonstrated periodic acid-Schiff (PAS) staining macrophages within the enteric mucosa of affected patients. This PAS positive material was shown to be due to the presence of a rod shaped bacteria (*Tropheryma whippelii*) which has recently been propagated in cell culture by coadministration of interleukin 4. The polymerase chain reaction may also be useful diagnostically in serum and CSF samples. Postmortem studies suggest that the nervous system is involved in most cases but clinical manifestations occur in only 10% of patients. The neurological manifestations of Whipple's disease are protean and may occur in isolation, leading to diagnostic difficulty. The CSF can be unremarkable but an increased protein level, pleocytosis and positive oligoclonal bands also occur. MRI may be normal but generalised atrophy or white matter lesions on T2 weighting with gadolinium enhancement have been described. If there are white matter lesions, these show a predilection for the temporal lobes, brainstem and hypothalamus. A slowly progressive dementia is the commonest neurological complication of Whipple's disease, often in combination with signs of brainstem and hypothalamic dysfunction, as in our case. An unusual movement disorder known as oculomasticatory myorhythmia is specifically associated with Whipple's disease. This is characterised by rhythmic convergence of the eyes and synchronous contraction of the masticatory muscles with an associated vertical gaze palsy. Other CNS features include ataxia, seizures, myoclonus, pyramidal signs and a reversible parkinsonian syndrome. Peripheral nervous system involvement has also been reported including a demyelinating neuropathy or myopathy. In the pre-antibiotic era Whipple's disease was uniformly fatal. Antibiotics which display good CNS penetration (such as co-trimoxazole) in combination with penicillin or tetracycline may lead to considerable clinical improvement. Prolonged courses are needed and relapse is common.

Reference

Wills AJ, Hovell CJ. Neurological complications of enteric disease. *Gut* 1996;**39**:501–4.

CASE 32

History	A 55-year-old woman developed migraine 10 years previously. This was treated successfully with pizotifen. Following this she became rather depressed and forgetful. At the age of 49 she developed a sudden onset of weakness affecting the left lower limb, with incomplete recovery. Three years later the left sided weakness deteriorated suddenly, with additional involvement of the upper limb. Subsequent to this her gait and cognitive function deteriorated in a stepwise fashion and she developed urinary frequency, hesitancy and occasional incontinence. She was a non-smoker. Her father and paternal uncle had suffered with a similar illness.

Examination

The patient was partially orientated and had poor short-term memory. Her gait was hesitant and characterised by small shuffling steps. She was slow to turn. Cranial nerve examination was normal. She had bilateral palmomental reflexes. Examination of the peripheral nervous system revealed bilateral lower limb pyramidal weakness with increased tone and sustained clonus. Reflexes were pathologically brisk with bilaterally extensor plantar responses. There were no sensory abnormalities. Her blood pressure was 115/70 mmHg and there were no carotid bruits or cardiac murmurs.

Investigations

MRI of the brain demonstrated generalised atrophy and diffuse signal abnormalities within the white matter, including subcortical and brainstem structures. There was additional involvement of the basal ganglia. MRI of the cord was normal. CSF was normal. Routine haematology and biochemistry, including detailed clotting screen, were normal. Cerebral and carotid angiography were normal. Psychosomatic testing revealed evidence of global cognitive impairment, but the patient performed particularly poorly on tests sensitive to frontal dysfunction.

Diagnosis Cerebral autosomal dominant arteriopathy with subcortical infarcts and leukoencephalopathy (CADASIL)

Commentary by Professor Richard S J Frackowiak

This woman has a typical presentation of CADASIL. There is a family history, compatible with autosomal dominant transmission. The disease has been mapped

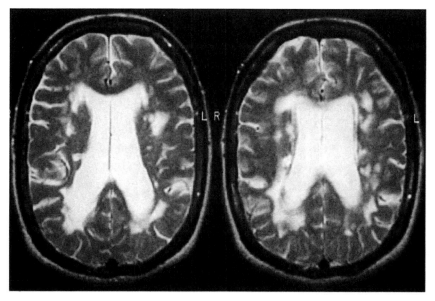

Figure 22 CADASIL. T2 weighted MRI scan showing diffuse atrophy and high signal change.

onto chromosome 19 and autosomal dominant transmission was confirmed from study of a large French family in 1991. The responsible gene has now been identified and a mutation in notch 3 demonstrated. The exact mechanism whereby the faulty gene causes the particular neurovascular phenotype is unclear. The onset is typically in mid-adulthood with migraine followed by progression secondary to multiple subcortical infarcts. The patient may present with transient ischaemic attacks as well as strokes. The MRI usually shows prominent signal change in the basal ganglia and white matter (Figure 22). The genetic abnormalities can be used as a diagnostic tool. The pathological picture is of an arteriopathy resulting in small deep infarcts and leukoencephalopathy. There are often haematomas which may be subcortical or may occur in the internal capsule. They also occur in the basal ganglia and brain stem, although the cortex is usually spared. The vascular wall is thickened by sudanophilic material in the media, which damages the smooth muscle cells. The same material may be found in muscle and skin vessels of some patients. There are pathological distinctions from amyloid and the changes in arteriosclerotic angiopathy. It is not yet clear whether muscle or skin biopsy can be used diagnostically. Treatment is supportive.

Reference

Chabriat H, Vahedi K, Iba-Zizen MT, *et al*. Clinical Spectrum of CADASIL: a study of 7 families. *Lancet* 1995;**346**:934–9.

CASE 33

History   A 39-year-old man had emigrated to the UK from India 2 years previously. He gave a 4-month history of burning paraesthesiae with subsequent numbness affecting his fingertips. He had also developed a scaly, dry red patch over his left cheek. He was otherwise fit and well. There was no family history of note and he drank 10 units of alcohol per week.

Examination

He had numerous scars over his fingers, an ulcer on the left heel and a number of diffuse hypopigmentary areas over the trunk. Cranial nerve examination was normal. There was weakness of finger abduction in the right hand and wasting of the first dorsal interosseous muscle. Reflexes were normal and plantar responses were flexor. There was patchy sensory loss affecting the limbs and trunk with additional involvement of both ears and the left cheek. The greater auricular and right ulnar nerves were enlarged.

Investigations

Nerve conduction studies demonstrated a demyelinating poyneuropathy with conduction block. Skin biopsy was normal.

Diagnosis   Tuberculoid leprosy

Commentary by Dr Kailash Bhatia

It is important to note that this patient is of Indian origin, and therefore is susceptible to mycobacterial infections. The different clinical forms of leprosy

109

are determined by immunological factors. In high cell-mediated immunity states causing tuberculoid or paucibacillary leprosy (Hansen's disease), hypopigmentary and hypoaesthetic skin patches occur over the face and trunk with an associated mononeuritis multiplex. The most commonly affected nerves are the greater auricular, ulnar and common peroneal nerves. In contrast, lepromatous or multibacillary leprosy can produce widespread symmetrical areas of anaesthesia and anhidrosis and a clinical picture resembling a distal polyneuropathy. However, in contrast with a typical polyneuropathy, sensation on the palms and soles is spared, as are the deep tendon reflexes, until late in the disease course. In this patient the long-standing scars and patchy sensory loss over the ears and cheeks can probably be attributed to tuberculoid leprosy which has caused thickening of the greater auricular and ulnar nerves. However, the recent history of burning paraesthesiae and the sensory loss affecting the limbs and trunk is unusual for tuberculoid leprosy. I wonder if this patient had developed an additional chronic inflammatory demyelinating polyneuropathy with conduction block, as suggested by the nerve conduction studies. Conduction blocks can occur in tuberculoid leprosy, but usually only at pressure points such as the elbow. It is important that the skin biopsy was taken from an area affected by hypopigmentation, although in tuberculoid leprosy the biopsy may be normal.

Reference

Swift TR, Sabin TD. Leprosy. In: Shakir RA, Newman PK, Poser CM, Eds. *Tropical Neurology*. London: WB Saunders; 1996:151–66.

CASE 34

History	A 16-year-old boy had an uneventful birth and delivery. The initial Apgar score was 9/10. He was noted to have initial feeding difficulties although his height and weight were normal. His head circumference was below the ninety-fifth centile. His motor milestones were delayed and he was unable to walk until the age of 4 years. In addition, his cognitive milestones were less severely delayed. At the age of 5 years he had his first epileptic seizure. His seizures continued throughout childhood and responded only partially to treatment. His parents were unrelated and there was no family history of neurological disorders.

Examination

The patient was fair-haired and blue-eyed. His secondary sexual characteristics were delayed. He was brachycephalic with a prominent occipital ridge. He was dysmorphic with an elfin face and prominent jaw. He laughed excessively during the examination. His language skills were rather poor, although comprehension seemed relatively preserved. The gait was abnormal with a flexed posture and elevation of the upper limbs. He had poor motor control with irregular jerking movements affecting all four limbs. There were no other neurological abnormalities.

Investigations

A CT brain scan confirmed brachycephaly but was otherwise normal. An EEG demonstrated three unusual features. There was large amplitude rhythmic 200–300 µvolt activity with superimposed multifocal spikes. In addition there was 2–3 Hz generalised slow activity that was maximal anteriorly, also intermingled with spikes. The third feature was semi-random posterior discharges noted on eye closure and associated with leg jerking.

> **Diagnosis**   Angelman's syndrome

Commentary by Dr Robert A H Surtees

Angelman's syndrome has five characteristic features: delayed development from early infancy; a movement disorder; suggestive facial features; unprovoked laughter; and specific EEG features.

The cognitive deficit is usually severe but is non-progressive, and speech is particularly affected. Both verbal comprehension and expression are extremely delayed and rarely progress beyond that of a normal two-year old. The movement disorder is best described as a jerky ataxia with frequent hand-clapping stereotypies; walking is achieved in most patients but is late and may be lost later in life. Suggestive facial features evolve with time and include a prominent lower jaw, wide mouth and thin upper lip. Patients have a happy disposition and may have bursts of laughter (which may not be euphoric). There are three EEG features, developing after 6–9 months of age, that are suggestive of Angelman's syndrome: runs of high-amplitude rhythmic delta activity with a frontal emphasis; runs of high-amplitude rhythmic theta activity; and runs of rhythmic sharp theta activity posteriorly facilitated by eye closure. Seizures occur in virtually all patients; the mean age of onset is 2 years and most will have developed seizures by 4 years. Commonly episodes of non-convulsive (and more rarely convulsive) status epilepticus occur. The epilepsy can be intractable to medical treatment but ameliorates with age. Angelman's syndrome is one of the best examples of a disorder where genetic imprinting is important. The 'Angelman gene' appears to be a maternally derived ubiquitin ligase encoding gene *UBE3A/E6-AP* on the long arm of chromosome 15. This gene is silenced in the paternally derived chromosome 15 in the brain by methylation under the control of the 'imprinting centre'. Most cases of Angelman's syndrome are sporadic and caused by *de novo* maternal deletions at *15q11–q13* which can be detected cytogenetically by fluorescent in situ hybridisation (FISH). A few percent are caused by paternal uniparental disomy, and a similar number by 'imprinter mutations' where the maternal gene is silenced. Both of these can be detected by the methylation pattern of *15q11–q13*. Of the remainder, point mutations of *UBE3A/E6-AP* have been found in a proportion.

Reference

Clayton-Smith J. Angelman's syndrome. *Arch Dis Child* 1992;**67**:889–91.

CASE 35

History	An 18-year-old university student presented with an upper respiratory tract infection with associated pyrexia, malaise and anorexia. One week later she developed severe constipation with abdominal pain and was prescribed trimethoprim and an enema for a presumed urinary tract infection. Two days later she began vomiting. The abdominal pain continued unabated and she complained of headaches. She became agitated and confused with associated diplopia and was admitted to hospital. Her clinical condition did not improve on intravenous antibiotic therapy and she suffered two generalised tonic–clonic seizures which were controlled with intravenous diazepam. After initial improvement, her conscious level deteriorated and she was transferred to the National Hospital. The patient's mother had undergone an appendicectomy for acute abdominal pain with normal histology.

Examination

On examination, the patient was agitated and apyrexial. She was tachycardic (120 beats per minute) and hypertensive (140/110 mmHg). She had generalised abdominal tenderness without rebound. Bowel sounds were present. The rest of the general examination was normal with no neck stiffness or rash. She was able to count fingers with either eye but the pupillary reactions were normal. Fundoscopy was normal. There were no lateralising neurological signs. Both plantar responses were flexor.

Investigations

Results of the full blood count are shown in Table 5. Urea and electrolytes, liver function tests and glucose levels were normal, but there was hyponatraemia (Na

Table 5 Haematological investigations	
haemoglobin	9.6 g/dl
MCV	79.6 fl
iron	5.6 µmol/l (normal = 12–30 µmol/l)
total iron binding capacity (TIBC)	90 µmol/l (normal = 45–80 µmol/l)
ferritin	normal

127 mmol/l) and a raised ALT of 175 IU/l (normal range = 7–56 IU/l). Ammonia and lactate levels were normal. The creatine kinase level was 22893 IU/l (normal range <160 IU/l). CRP and ESR, lead levels and CSF were normal. Urinary porphyrins measured 930 nmol/l (normal range 0–320 nmol/l), and urinary porphobilinogen measured 165.3 µmol/l (normal range 0–8.8 µmol/l). Erythrocyte hydroxymethylbilane synthase (formerly porphobilinogen deaminase) measured 20 nmol uroporphyrin/ml red cells/hour (normal range 20–42). Faecal porphyrins were normal. The EEG showed generalised slow waves with intermittent sharp waves. An MRI scan of the brain showed bilateral occipital lobe high-signal change on T2 weighting (low signal on T1) involving cortical and subcortical structures. There was a minor degree of enhancement with gadolinium. MRV was normal.

Diagnosis   Acute intermittent porphyria

Commentary by Dr John M Land

Acute intermittent porphyria (AIP) is an autosomal dominant inherited deficiency of haem biosynthesis in which patients and gene carriers have a 50% deficiency of PBG deaminase. Ninety percent of those who inherit the gene defect remain asymptomatic throughout their lives. Women are more prone to acute attacks than men. Symptoms are rarely noted prior to puberty but may be related to menstruation and pregnancy. AIP may be precipitated by a number of drugs including oestrogens, barbiturates and alcohol. These are believed to increase the activity of the normally rate-limiting hepatic aminolaevulinic acid synthase, the enzyme immediately prior to PBG deaminase, in response to increased requirements for haem coenzyme by the drug detoxification system cytochrome P450. This effectively overwhelms the reduced PBG deaminase system and causes accumulation of PBG, and to a lesser extent ALA, which are excreted in the urine. Irregular meals and increased alcohol consumption were possibly contributory to this patient's acute presentation. Abdominal pain is an extremely common presenting symptom and patients are often mistakenly thought to have acute appendicitis. Mild hypertension and an isolated raised ALT is not uncommon, the latter reflecting hepatic involvement. Neurological complications occur in many patients. These include peripheral neuropathies, confusional states, seizures and coma. It is intriguing to speculate that the neurological presentation may reflect impaired cerebral oxidative energy metabolism secondary to brain mitochondrial cytochrome deficiencies. The MRI changes which are similar to those seen in mitochondrial encephalopathies would support this view. Photosensitivity is not a feature. Similar presentations to AIP are observed in hereditary tyrosinaemia and lead poisoning. The former is easily excluded on the basis of hepatic function and amino acid analysis. In lead poisoning porphobilinogen is not seen in the urine, suggesting that ALA may be the common toxic agent in AIP and lead poisoning. Interpretation of red cell enzymological studies requires great care in the presence of anaemia, as in this case, where the mean age of the cells is reduced. As cells age enzyme levels fall. Thus, patient results when compared to reference intervals derived from cells with an older mean age may appear normal or only marginally low. DNA studies provide the definitive diagnosis. Management including a high carbohydrate intake and avoidance of precipitant drugs is usually very successful. In this case the mother was subsequently shown to be affected, although she had only ever had one episode of abdominal pain and no neurological problems.

Reference

Gupta S, Dolwani S. Neurological complications of porphyria. *Postgrad Med J* 1996;**72:**631–2.

CASE 36

History	A 77-year-old man presented with a 5-week history of headache and diplopia. The headache had become progressively more severe and was mainly located over the occiput. It tended to wake him up in the early morning. His diplopia was worse on looking to the right; the images were separated in a horizontal plane. He had developed non-insulin-dependent diabetes 5 years previously but was otherwise well. He had been exposed to asbestos in the past and had smoked 50 cigarettes a day until 10 years previously.

Examination

General examination was normal. There was no finger clubbing. Neurologically, there was evidence of a right sixth nerve palsy with no other abnormalities.

Investigations

The full blood count was normal. ESR was 62 mm/hour. Routine biochemistry was normal. Protein electrophoresis demonstrated the presence of an IgG kappa paraprotein (14.5 g/l). The skeletal survey was normal. Chest X-ray showed consolidation in the left mid-zone with pleural thickening and a calcified plaque over the right diaphragm. A CT scan of the chest revealed a mass in the left upper lobe and associated mediastinal lymphadenopathy (Figure 23). A CT scan of the brain showed a soft tissue mass in the skull base involving the petrous temporal bone and clivus. Subsequently, bronchoscopy was performed. Cytological examination of the bronchoscopic specimen revealed the presence of a keratinising squamous cell carcinoma.

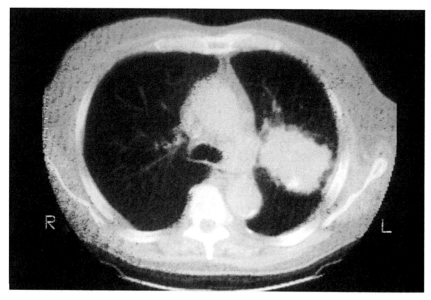

Figure 23 *Squamous cell carcinoma. CT scan of the thorax showing a mass in the left upper lobe.*

Diagnosis	Metastatic deposit at skull base probably arising from a squamous lung carcinoma.
	Coincidental benign monoclonal gammopathy

Commentary by Dr Adrian J Wills

The investigation of an isolated sixth nerve palsy is predominantly determined by the age of onset. In children, this may occur as a post viral phenomenon and has a good prognosis. In addition, chronic middle ear infections can be complicated by a petrositis extending to involve the fifth and seventh cranial nerves with associated deafness (Gradenigo's syndrome) or by a lateral sinus thrombosis with subsequent elevation of intracranial pressure and a sixth nerve palsy as a false localising sign. In all age groups, an abducens palsy may be seen following fractures of the temporal bone or skull base. In young adults, demyelination may rarely present in this fashion. In older patients, as in our case, an ischaemic or neoplastic aetiology is far more likely. Medical conditions which can present in this manner include diabetes, vasculitis (including giant cell arteritis), hypertension, herpes zoster and meningovascular syphilis. Myasthenia gravis is an exceedingly rare cause of an isolated sixth nerve palsy. Horizontal diplopia may also be the presenting symptom of nasopharyngeal carcinomas and tumours of the clivus such as chordomas. In our case the base of skull mass was not biopsied; it was thought to be more likely a secondary from the known bronchial primary rather than an isolated plasmacytoma. A number of solid tumours have a predilection to metastasise to the brain parenchyma, usually at the grey/white matter junction. These include lung, breast, renal and colonic tumours and melanomas. Patients usually present with headache and localising signs, although focal seizures may also occur. Tumours of the prostate and ovary and sarcomas rarely metastasise to the brain. A number of neoplasms classically metastasise to the leptomeninges including leukaemias, lymphomas, melanomas and breast tumours. These may cause a meningitic picture and can present a diagnostic challenge. Repeat CSF analysis coupled with contrast enhanced MRI scan are the investigations of choice. At postmortem, intracranial metastases can be demonstrated in 25% of cancer patients.

Reference

Posner JB. Intracranial metastases. In: Posner JB, Ed. *Neurologic Complications of Cancer.* Philadelphia: FA Davis; 1995:77–110.

CASE 37

<table>
<tr>
<td>History</td>
<td>A 29-year-old woman was well until 4 years previously when she developed loss of vision in the right eye with associated retro-orbital pain which was worse on eye movement. At worst the visual acuity in the affected eye was 6/60, improving back to 6/24 following steroid treatment. One year later, similar symptoms occurred in the same eye with improvement following treatment. At the age of 29 years she developed numbness commencing in the right forearm and gradually radiating to the trunk, with band-like sensory loss involving the lower dorsal region. Following this, both lower limbs became progressively weaker with associated hesitancy of micturition and constipation. In addition, she developed severe right retro-orbital pain with marked loss of visual acuity on that side (no perception of light). The rest of the history was unremarkable and there was no family history of neurological disorders.</td>
</tr>
</table>

Examination

General examination was normal. Visual acuity was 6/6 on the left with normal colour vision and perception of light only on the right. Both optic discs were pale (more marked on the right) with a right relative afferent pupillary defect. The eye movements and remaining cranial nerves were normal. Examination of the upper limbs was normal. There was a pyramidal weakness and increased tone affecting both lower limbs with sustained ankle clonus. Both plantar responses were extensor. There was diminished sensation involving all modalities with a level at T6. Cerebellar function was normal.

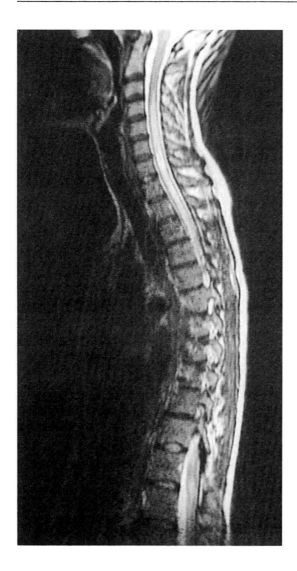

Figure 24 T2 weighted MRI scan of the cord demonstrating a long, high signal intrinsic lesion.

Investigations

Routine haematology and biochemistry were normal. Serum ACE level was normal. B_{12} levels, syphilis serology and ANF were normal or negative. The chest X-ray and MRI brain scan were normal. MRI of the cord showed a long, high signal intrinsic lesion extending from C3 to T7 with associated cord swelling (Figure 24). CSF analysis was abnormal with a raised protein level (1.1 g/l), six lymphocytes and positive oligoclonal bands.

Diagnosis   Devic's syndrome

Commentary by Professor David H Miller

There is controversy regarding the classification of Devic's syndrome. Some consider it to be a variant of multiple sclerosis, whereas others view it as a distinct disease entity. At the core of the syndrome is a monophasic or multiphasic illness with acute neurological episodes confined to the spinal cord and optic nerves. Sometimes specific causes, including systemic lupus erythematosis and acute disseminated encephalomyelitis are identified. It is also recognised in association with a previous history of tuberculosis. Undoubtedly, many patients with relapsing spinal cord and optic nerve symptoms merge into the picture of classical multiple sclerosis (MS). There does appear to be a small group of patients who nevertheless have a number of clinical and investigative findings that are distinct from MS. These include; severe complete myelitis, poor recovery from episodes of myelitis and optic neuritis, normal brain MRI, negative oligoclonal bands and extensive spinal swelling over many segments in the acute phase. The above patient illustrates some but not all of these features. Therapy is empirical. High-dose intravenous steroids are often used to treat acute relapses. It is not known whether immunomodulatory therapy modifies the long-term prognosis.

Reference

O'Riordan JL, Gallagher HL, Thompson AJ, *et al*. The clinical, cerebrospinal fluid and MRI findings in Devic's neuromyelitis optica. *J Neurol Neurosurg Psychiatry* 1996;**60**:382–7.

CASE 38

History	A 26-year-old woman was the product of a normal full-term delivery. Her initial cognitive and motor milestones were normal. She started having absence attacks at the age of 8 years and was given treatment with anticonvulsants. Three years later she was noted to be dragging her left leg when she walked, her left hand became increasingly clumsy and she developed a left facial weakness. In addition, she was noted to have involuntary jerking movements affecting her left sided limbs with frequent secondary generalisation. The seizures became intractable resulting in frequent hospital admissions for status epilepticus. Her cognitive function deteriorated and the left sided weakness became increasingly severe.

Examination

The patient had marked left hemiatrophy. Rhythmical jerking affecting the left foot was noted throughout the examination. Cranial nerve examination revealed a left inferior quadrantanopia and a left upper motor neurone facial weakness. There was a marked left hemiplegia with reflex asymmetry (left brisker than right). Both plantar responses were flexor. Sensory examination was unrevealing as she was rather drowsy and uncooperative.

Investigations

Routine haematology and biochemistry were normal. An MRI scan of the brain revealed a shrunken right cerebral hemisphere with enlargement of the right lateral ventricle. In addition, the left cerebellar hemisphere was also atrophic. An EEG was grossly abnormal with low-amplitude slow waves and intermittent periodic sharp waves over the right hemisphere. CSF analysis was normal.

> **Diagnosis**   Rasmussen's encephalitis

Commentary by Professor Simon D Shorvon

Rasmussen's encephalitis was first described in 1955, and there have been about 100 cases reported since in the literature. This case is characteristic in many ways. The age of onset after normal early development is typical, as is the presentation with epilepsy and the subsequent development of a slowly progressive hemiplegia and cognitive dysfunction. The epilepsy is often severe in this condition, and episodes of status are usual. Many patients have periods of Epilepsia Partialis Continua (EPC) and this was a feature noted here. The aetiology of Rasmussen's encephalitis has not been established. Histologically, the condition has the appearance of an encephalitis, and the involvement of a number of infectious agents has been suggested on the basis of polymerase chain reactions and in situ hybridisation (including cytomegalovirus, herpes simplex, Epstein–Barr virus and herpes virus 6). However, none has been consistently found. Inclusion bodies and viral particles have not been identified. Attempts to transmit the disorder by cerebral inoculation of brain biopsy material and to isolate a virus by cell culture have failed. Recently, antibodies to the GluR3 subunit of the glutamate receptor were detected in two patients, but this too does not seem to be a consistent finding. In the absence of a clear-cut aetiology, medical treatment is empirical and is generally unsatisfactory. Immunosuppression and antiviral therapy have been attempted without consistent success. The epilepsy should be treated with conventional antiepileptic therapy. Hemispherectomy (or at least a wide excision of the area affected by the encephalitis) will halt the progression of the condition in most cases. However, hemispherectomy causes significant deficit, and as the condition has a tendency to stop progressing (usually after 5–10 years), the timing of operation is often difficult to decide.

Reference

Hart YM, Andermann F, Fish DR. Chronic encephalitis and epilepsy in adults and adolescents: a variety of Rasmussen's syndrome. *Neurol* 1997;**48**:418–24.

CASE 39

History	A 19-year-old woman had been born in the UK but had made frequent trips to Pakistan. She was well until 4 years previously when she developed tiredness, weight loss and secondary amenorrhea. Six months later she complained of intermittent arthralgia. One year after the onset of her symptoms she became rapidly drowsy, lapsed into a coma and was admitted to hospital in Pakistan. CSF analysis at that stage was abnormal with 120 white cells (80% lymphocytes) and she was given intravenous acyclovir and quadruple antituberculous chemotherapy. She recovered slowly and continued on rifampicin, isoniazid and pyrazinamide for 1 year. Two months after cessation of the antibiotics she developed a low grade fever and abdominal pain. CSF analysis was again abnormal with a protein level of 6.2 g/l, glucose level of 0.7 mmol/l (plasma level was 5.1 mmol/l) and an elevated white count of 132 cells (36% lymphocytes). She was administered antituberculous treatment again and partially improved. Subsequently she developed profound deafness.

Examination

The patient was alert and orientated with mild meningism and a pyrexia (38°C). The remainder of the general and neurological exam was normal apart from bilateral severe sensorineural hearing loss.

Investigations

Routine haematology and biochemistry were normal. Blood cultures were negative. *Brucella* serology by ELISA revealed an IgG titre of 640, the IgM titre 80, the complement fixation test titre was >256. MRI investigation of the brain was normal. Following a change in antibiotics (doxycycline, septrin and rifampicin) the CSF analysis was repeated and showed an elevated protein level of 1.36 g/l, 10 white cells (lymphocytes) and positive oligoclonal bands with fewer bands in the serum . CSF culture for acid-fast bacilli was negative.

Diagnosis   Neurobrucellosis

Commentary by Dr Raad A W Shakir

The differential diagnosis of a chronic meningitis is not straightforward. Treatment for tuberculosis was instituted in this case purely on the grounds of chronic lymphocytic meningitis. The recurrence of symptoms after cessation of anti-tuberculous treatment is intriguing. Rifampicin was used as part of the treatment but this was probably insufficient to eradicate completely the intracellular *Brucella*. We do not know which *Brucella* species was isolated and it would have been appropriate to do a bone marrow culture although this is not positive in all cases, especially in a patient who has been partially treated. We also have no information on whether there was any evidence of systemic involvement such as sacroiliac joint arthritis. A bone scan would have been useful in this context to delineate any 'hot' areas in the lower lumbar spine or elsewhere. Culture of *Brucella* is possible in only 25% of proven neurobrucellosis cases and so one has to rely on serological tests. The CSF ELISA tends to be more specific, especially if there is an elevated IgM titre. PCR of the CSF has also been reported to be diagnostically useful. From the clinical point of view, the patient had features of a chronic meningitis associated with bilateral deafness which is quite common in neurobrucellosis. Oligoclonal bands are known to occur in this illness. The protean manifestations of neurobrucellosis have been known for a long time and a high index of clinical suspicion, coupled with performance of the appropriate serological tests is the only way of arriving at a diagnosis. Treatment consists of a combination of rifampicin, doxycycline and co-trimoxazole which should continue for a minimum of 3 months and a maximum of 6 months. Repeated lumbar puncture is essential to demonstrate normalisation of CSF constituents. In chronic neurobrucellosis, whether characterised by meningeal or parenchymal involvement, improvement of neurological deficits such as deafness is unlikely.

Reference

Shakir RA. Brucellosis. In: Shakir RA, Newman PK, Poser CM, Eds. *Tropical Neurology*. London: WB Saunders; 1996:167–81.

CASE 40

History   A 61-year-old woman had developed carcinoma of the cervix 30 years previously and had been treated with radiotherapy. At the age of 51 years she presented with bowel obstruction secondary to a rectal stricture. This was corrected surgically but 3 years later she required a colostomy because of severe proctitis which was concluded to be related to the previous radiotherapy. At the age of 57 years she developed back pain radiating to the right leg which had a burning quality. This became progressively more severe with associated right lower limb weakness and wasting. She also complained of urinary frequency and stress incontinence. She had non-insulin-dependent diabetes with onset at the age of 56 years. One year later she developed ureteric obstruction necessitating a right nephrectomy.

Examination

Neurological abnormalities were confined to the lower limbs. The right calf, hamstring and gluteal muscles were wasted. There was global weakness of the right lower limb with predominant involvement of the hip flexors and ankle evertors. The right knee and ankle jerks were absent. Both plantar responses were flexor. Sensation was reduced over the L3–S2 dermatomes on the right.

Investigations

An MRI scan of the lumbar spine showed a left lateral disc bar at L5/S1 with lateral displacement of the left L5 nerve root. CT examination of the pelvis was normal. An EMG demonstrated marked denervation in S1 and L5 innervated muscles on the right with lesser involvement of the remaining lumbar myotomes. In addition, there were milder denervation changes in the L5/S1 myotomes on the left. There was additional mild lumbar paraspinal muscle denervation. No myokymia was seen.

Diagnosis Radiation lumbosacral plexopathy

Commentary by Dr Adrian J Wills and Dr John W Scadding

The clinician may be faced with the often difficult task of distinguishing radiation induced plexopathy from cancerous invasion. Doses of radiation exceeding 6000 rads are particularly associated with subsequent neurological complications but there is no relationship between the latency of onset and total dose administered. This problem is compounded by the fact that the latency between a course of radiotherapy treatment and the subsequent development of neurological symptoms may vary from 3 months to over 20 years. A helpful diagnostic pointer is the occurrence of pain which is almost invariably present in tumour plexopathies (98% of patients) but less likely in radiation induced cases (50%). In neoplastic invasion of the lumbosacral plexus the pain is followed at an interval of weeks or months by weakness, parasthaesiae, numbness, and incontinence or impotence in a minority (less than 10%). Examination may indicate either an upper or lower plexopathy but there are eventually signs of a pan-plexopathy. In the great majority of patients the plexopathy is unilateral. The tumours most often causing lumbosacral neoplastic invasion are colorectal cancer, sarcomas and genitourinary cancers. By contrast, in radiation lumbosacral plexopathy, the earliest symptoms are usually weakness and numbness in one or both legs. Most patients eventually develop bilateral symptoms and signs. Weakness and sensory loss is diffuse in about half of the patients, predominantly distal in most of the remainder and predominantly proximal (L2 to L4) in a small minority. Bladder or bowel symptoms may be present but are usually due to the direct effect of radiation rather than neurogenic in origin. In the upper limbs, the presence of lymphoedema or upper trunk involvement is also highly suggestive of radiation induced damage (the lower trunk may be protected from ionising damage by the clavicle and its shorter course). In contrast, metastatic brachial plexopathies preferentially affect the lower trunk and an associated Horner's syndrome is far more likely to occur (54% versus 14%).

130

An EMG may be particularly useful in showing myokymic discharges in about half of the radiation induced cases (this virtually never occurs in cancerous infiltration), indicating additional nerve root involvement. In lumbosacral plexopathy a rectal examination is mandatory (a pelvic exam should also be performed in women). Additional investigations which may be useful include MRI of the plexus (which is normal in radiation induced cases), CT of the pelvis and occasionally CSF examination. The pathology of radiation plexopathy is a progressive perineurial and endoneurial fibrosis with vascular obliteration leading to ischaemic nerve damage. There is also evidence that direct radiation damage occurs to myelin sheaths and axons. The pathological changes are usually relentlessly progressive, leading to severe disability in a majority of patients over several years. In this particular patient the pain and unilateral involvement pointed to possible malignant infiltration, whereas the long latency before symptom onset favoured a radiation plexopathy. However, in most cases, survival after tumour recurrence is of the order of 2 years whereas this patient's symptoms had been present for 5 years, suggesting radiation induced damage.

Reference

Thomas JE, Cascino TL, Earle JD, et al. Differential diagnosis between radiation and tumour plexopathy of the pelvis. *Neurol* 1985;**35**:1–7.

CASE 41

History A 59-year-old man was well until 3 years previously when he developed episodes of neurological disturbance. The attacks were characterised by pins and needles affecting the right hand followed by speech arrest which would last for up to 2 minutes, occurring twice daily. He was prescribed aspirin but this did not alter the frequency of attacks. He had chronic airflow limitation and continued to smoke but was otherwise well. Over the past 10 years he had noticed increasing numbers of dark blue facial lesions which bled when scratched.

Examination

The patient had multiple bluish lesions over his face, arms and trunk. These did not blanch with pressure. He was rather obese and auscultation of the chest revealed widespread polyphonic wheezes. The rest of the general and neurological exam was normal.

Investigations

Chest X-ray and EEG were normal. An MRI scan of the brain showed multiple areas of haemosiderin staining, some of which contained a high signal centre. These were primarily situated in the right cerebellar hemisphere, right inferior frontal lobe and left parietal lobe and cingulate gyrus. Radiologically, these had the appearance of multiple cavernomas. One of his skin lesions was biopsied and revealed changes consistent with capillary haemangiomata.

Diagnosis Blue rubber bleb nevus syndrome presenting with frontal lobe seizures

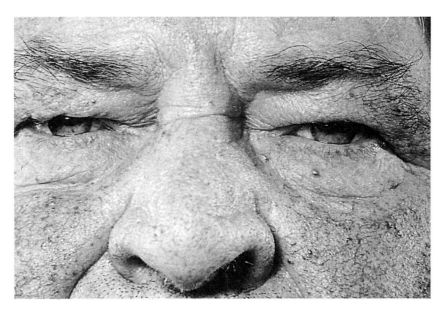

Figure 25 Blue rubber bleb syndrome. Characteristic facial appearance.

Commentary by Dr Adrian J Wills

The blue rubber bleb nevus syndrome was first described by Bean in 1958. It is an uncommon viscero-cutaneous haemangiomatosis in which scattered, bluish, rubbery naevi occur on the body surface (Figure 25). These are often noticeable from birth. In a few cases the syndrome may be familial. The lesions tend to bleed easily and may present with gastrointestinal haemorrhage or iron deficiency anaemia secondary to more chronic blood loss. Angiomata have been documented in several organs including the lungs, liver, peritoneum and skeletal muscle. Central nervous system (CNS) involvement is rare. Satya-Murti and co-workers described the case of a 19-year-old man who presented with a progressive cerebellar syndrome secondary to multiple brainstem haemangiomas. However, focal seizures have also been described, as in our case. MRI typically shows high signal change on T2 weighting secondary to either low

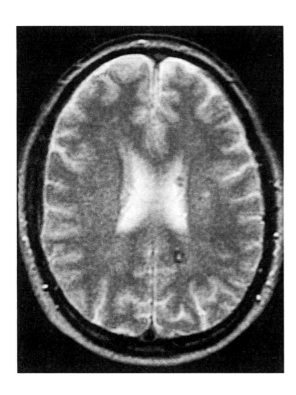

Figure 26 Cavernous angioma in blue rubber bleb syndrome. T2 weighted MRI scan demonstrating haemosiderin (low density) surrounding a high signal centre.

blood flow or thrombosis (Figure 26). The lesions may calcify, which can be demonstrated easily on CT scans. The main differential diagnosis is hereditary haemorrhagic telangiectasia. The skin lesions may be treated with laser therapy. CNS angiomas may be surgically resected or alternatively lesioned radiosurgically. In the main, a conservative approach to management is adopted unless there are intractable seizures or a progressive neurological deficit. Our patient's seizures responded well to anticonvulsants. Most of the neurological cases reported in the literature are associated with a poor prognosis.

Reference

Satya-Murti S, Navada S, Eames F. Central nervous system involvement in blue rubber bleb nevus syndrome. *Arch Neurol* 1986;**43**:1184–6.

135

CASE 42

History	A 16-year-old boy had developed exertional cyanosis with limited exercise tolerance 6 years previously. He also noticed attacks of neurological disturbance consisting of left sided paraesthesiae and numbness lasting a few seconds, occurring up to four times daily. On occasions following these episodes he would be unable to move his left hand for several minutes. At the age of 15 years, following an episode of sensory disturbance, he was witnessed to have a generalised tonic–clonic seizure. Following this he had a number of other generalised seizures and was prescribed carbamazepine with good effect. He had previously suffered with recurrent nose bleeds but there was no other relevant past medical history. His paternal grandmother also had a history of recurrent epistaxes and died following a subarachnoid haemorrhage. His father also had recurrent epistaxes.

Examination

The general and neurological examination was normal with no evidence of cutaneous telangiectases.

Investigations

A CT brain scan showed a serpiginous increase in signal over the right frontal parietal area. There was also a smaller high-density left temporal lesion. Cerebral angiography confirmed the presence of a large arteriovenous malformation (AVM) lying towards the convexity of the right cerebral hemisphere and supplied by branches of the right middle and anterior cerebral arteries. A second AVM was also demonstrated filling from posterior medial choroidal branches on the left.

> **Diagnosis** Multiple cerebral and pulmonary arteriovenous malformations secondary to hereditary haemorrhagic telangiectasia

Commentary by Professor Richard S J Frackowiak

This 16-year-old boy presents with a genetic disorder of vessels that affected a grandmother and probably his father. He has a hereditary telangiectasia and arteriovenous malformations (AVMs) which are the most frequent abnormality of the intracranial circulation in childhood. The combination of the two is rare. The AVMs tend to be congenital lesions and it is more common for them to become symptomatic in the third or fourth decade of life. Haemorrhage is the most common presentation. In this instance the patient presented with symptoms of heart failure followed by transient neurological events and subsequent epilepsy, presumably secondary to a space-occupying effect of the AVMs or to secondary ischaemic damage. In this patient's case the difficulty lay in the fact that his life was probably more threatened by pulmonary shunts causing arterial desaturation than the cerebral lesions themselves. Therapy is a combination of surgical resection and/or interventional radiology and can be very successful in adolescents. Pulmonary AVMs require their own treatment, usually with embolisation. In general, intracranial vascular malformations can be divided into four groups; AVMs, capillary malformations or telangiectasia (this patient had a combination of these two), venous malformations and cavernous angiomas. The latter are often called cryptic angiomas as they are rarely revealed by angiographic studies and manifest as haemorrhages.

Reference

Ter-Berg JWM, Dippel DW, Habbema JD, *et al.* Unruptured intracranial arteriovenous malformations with hereditary haemorrhagic telangiectasia; Neurosurgical treatment or not? *Acta Neurochirurgica* 1993;**121**:34–42.

CASE 43

History	A 51-year-old man had noticed paraesthesiae affecting his fingertips 1 year previously. This was initially intermittent but became continuous. Six months later he noticed that his legs were stiff and this symptom became progressively more severe. His exercise tolerance deteriorated secondary to lower limb weakness. He also developed paraesthesiae in his feet and a band-like sensation across the lower abdomen. He had noticed no symptoms of autonomic dysfunction apart from a loss of erections over the previous year. At the age of 25 years he had developed pulmonary tuberculosis and had received antibiotics for 12 months. His mother had died of leukaemia at the age of 78 years and his maternal grandmother, uncle and aunt had all developed anaemia in adult life. He was a smoker and drank 30 units of alcohol per week. He had noticed some problems with his memory and concentration, leading to employment difficulties, and had been prescribed antidepressants without benefit.

Examination

The patient was pale with moderate conjunctival pallor. There were numerous spider naevi over his chest but no other stigmata of chronic liver disease. An ejection systolic murmur was clearly heard over the anterior chest wall with no carotid radiation. Cranial nerve and upper limb examination was unremarkable. In the lower limbs, tone was increased in a pyramidal fashion with mild weakness of hip flexion (grade 4+). Clonus could not be elicited at the knee or ankle. Knee reflexes were pathologically brisk, ankle jerks depressed and both plantar responses were extensor. Sensory examination revealed marked loss of joint position and vibration sense in the lower limbs with a rather patchy loss of light touch and pinprick sensation. His gait was spastic and Romberg's test was

Table 6 Haematological and biochemical investigations	
haemoglobin	10.1 g/dl
MCV	145 fl
platelets	5127 × 10⁹/l
serum B₁₂	53 ng/l (normal = 223–1132 ng/l)
Schilling test part 1	4.6% (normal range 14–40%)
Schilling test part 2	9.6% (normal range 14–40%)
ratio –	2.1 (normal range 0.7–1.2)

clearly positive. He had mild heel–shin ataxia but no upper limb ataxia and no involuntary movements.

Investigations

Results of haematological tests are shown in Table 6. The blood film showed poikilocytes, spherocytes and hypersegmented neutrophils. Urea and electrolytes, liver function tests, blood glucose and thyroid function tests were normal. Tests for autoantibodies, including gastric parietal and antiendomysial antibodies were negative. The test for intrinsic factor antibodies was positive. Red cell folate levels were normal. MRI of the cord was normal. Nerve conduction studies and EMG were compatible with a sensory peripheral neuropathy. Central motor conduction times were prolonged on recording from the lower limbs and normal in the upper limbs. Somatosensory evoked potentials were absent from both posterior tibial nerves and abnormal in the upper limbs consistent with delayed conduction in the large fibre central sensory pathway.

Diagnosis   Subacute combined degeneration secondary to pernicious anaemia

140

Commentary by Professor P K Thomas

A neurological presentation of vitamin B_{12} deficiency is currently uncommon, as a diagnosis is usually made when the individual develops a macrocytic anaemia. Although the diagnosis here is given as subacute combined degeneration of the cord, the neurological manifestations were clearly more widespread with symptoms related to involvement of the peripheral nerves and spinal cord and also of cognitive dysfunction. The patient's initial symptoms consisted of paraesthesiae in his fingers, presumably due to a sensory neuropathy; this was confirmed later by nerve conduction studies. Lower limb paraesthesiae developed subsequently. It is a feature of neuropathy related to vitamin B_{12} deficiency that the symptoms may begin in the upper limbs. Lhermitte's phenomenon may occur; this is probably related to stretching of the cervical spinal cord or roots on neck flexion. Spinal cord involvement was indicated in this patient by the presence of pyramidal signs in the legs, including extensor plantar responses. This accounted for his complaint of difficulty in walking. A motor peripheral neuropathy is not a feature of vitamin B_{12} deficiency. The sensory loss predominantly affected joint position and vibration sense. In view of the electrophysiological findings, this was probably due to a combination of a large fibre sensory neuropathy and posterior column dysfunction. In the early stages of subacute combined degeneration, sensory nerve action potentials may be normal but spinal somatosensory evoked potentials are delayed, indicating early damage to the ascending fibres in the posterior columns. Prognosis for recovery in subacute combined degeneration has to be guarded. In those patients in whom the manifestations consist predominantly of a sensory neuropathy, improvement on vitamin B_{12} replacement can be satisfactory, but it is less pronounced in patients who mainly show a myelopathy. The mechanism of neurological damage from vitamin B_{12} deficiency has been discussed by Thomas and Griffin (1995).

Reference

Thomas PK, Griffin JW. Neuropathies predominantly affecting motor or sensory function. In: Asbury AK, Thomas PK, Eds. *Peripheral Nerve Disorders 2*. Oxford: Butterworth Heinemann; 1995:59–94.

CASE 44

History	A 71-year-old woman presented with a 9-month history of severe paroxysmal left retro-orbital pain. The pain would last from 60 to 90 seconds and was occasionally but not consistently triggered by chewing or eating without being affected by other tactile stimuli. She had also noticed that the attacks were precipitated by driving through shafts of sunlight indicating some degree of flicker sensitivity. The attacks would occur every 10 minutes throughout the day and night and had been fairly persistent during the 9-month period. At worst, she could have up to 25 attacks in an hour. Associated symptoms included ipsilateral lacrimation, conjunctival suffusion and nasal stuffiness. There was no associated nausea or vomiting and no visual symptoms. She was not sensitive to light or sound during bouts and there was no effect of head movements. She had a past history of hypothyroidism and depression. She was taking thyroxine but no other medications. There was no family history of migraine or other neurological disorders. Indomethacin had previously been prescribed without benefit.

Examination

General and neurological examination was entirely normal. During an attack her left eye was noted to lacrimate and she developed marked conjunctival hyperaemia.

Investigations

MRI of the brain was normal.

> **Diagnosis** Short-lasting unilateral neuralgiform pain with conjunctival
> injection and tearing (SUNCT syndrome)

Commentary by Professor Peter J Goadsby

Short-lasting unilateral neuralgiform headache with conjunctival injection and tearing (SUNCT) is a remarkable syndrome that is classified between paroxysmal hemicrania and trigeminal neuralgia in terms of the length of attacks. Most reported cases are seen in men, with a male:female ratio of 17:4. The pain occurs in paroxysms that last between 5 and 250 seconds, although two patients have been described where attacks lasted up to 2 hours. Although patients may have as many as 30 episodes an hour, five to six attacks an hour is more usual. The frequency and length of attacks distinguishes this syndrome from cluster headache. A systematic study of attack frequency demonstrated a mean of 28 attacks per day with a range of 6 to 77. The conjunctival injection seen with SUNCT is often the most prominent autonomic feature, although tearing may also be very obvious. Other associated autonomic stigmata include sweating of the forehead or rhinorrhoea. The length of attacks and associated autonomic features distinguish this condition from trigeminal neuralgia. The attacks may become bilateral, but the most severe pain remains unilateral. Most cases have some associated precipitating factors, which include mechanical movements of the neck. There have been three reported patients with secondary SUNCT syndromes. The first two patients had ipsilateral cerebellopontine angle arteriovenous malformations diagnosed on MRI. The third patient had a cavernous hemangioma of the brainstem seen only on MRI. A posterior fossa lesion causing otherwise typical SUNCT has also been noted in human immunodeficiency virus/acquired immunodeficiency syndrome. These cases highlight the need for cranial MRI in investigating secondary SUNCT. SUNCT is remarkably refractory to treatment. Most drugs used in the treatment of other short-lasting headaches are not beneficial in SUNCT apart from verapamil, which may be helpful in high dose. Indomethacin is not useful in SUNCT, a fact which can differentiate this syndrome from paroxysmal hemicrania.

Reference

Goadsby PJ, Lipton RB. A review of paroxysmal hemicranias, SUNCT syndrome and other short-lasting headaches with autonomic features, including new cases. *Brain* 1997;**120**:193–209.

144

CASE 45

History	A 51-year-old Turkish man had been well until 3 weeks previously. He then developed headache, photophobia, myalgia and vomiting. He went to his local Casualty Department were he was noted to have meningism but no fever. Five days later he developed a progressive left hemiplegia associated with a diminished level of consciousness. He was admitted to hospital and found to be drowsy and pyrexial. His pupils were asymmetric (right larger than left) and he had an internuclear ophthalmoplegia. His left sided weakness had a pyramidal pattern and the left plantar response was extensor. Over the next 24 hours his neurological status deteriorated with a diminishing level of consciousness and the development of a fixed right pupil, generalised hyperreflexia and bilateral extensor plantar responses. He developed respiratory distress and was intubated and ventilated. He had previously been fit and well apart from recurrent bouts of anterior uveitis. His son had suffered with recurrent oral ulceration and a deep venous thrombosis with no apparent precipitants.

Examination

The patient was pyrexial (38°C) with moderate neck stiffness. There was no evidence of a rash or purpura. He had pharyngeal ulceration. Heart sounds were normal. He was obtunded but the doll's eye manoeuvre was normal. His pupils reacted sluggishly to light. Corneal reflexes were preserved and he coughed on suction. Tone was increased in a pyramidal fashion in the limbs, reflexes were pathologically brisk and both plantar responses were extensor.

Investigations

Routine haematology was normal. ESR was 70 mm/hour, and CRP was 29 mg/l. Urea, electrolytes and glucose levels were normal. Liver function tests were normal apart from a raised ALT (75 IU/l) and γGT (200 IU/l). Blood cultures were negative. The autoimmune profile, including ANCA was negative. Serological tests for Syphilis and Lyme disease were negative. Serum ACE level were normal. CSF analysis showed 10 lymphocytes, a protein level of 0.54 g/dl, glucose level of 4.6 mmol/l (plasma 6.8 mmol/l) and positive oligoclonal bands (matched with serum). MRI of the brain demonstrated high signal abnormalities on T2 weighting (low signal on T1) in the pons and midbrain extending to the internal capsules bilaterally. This was more marked on the right and the pons and midbrain were swollen. The right pontine and midbrain lesions were seen to patchily enhance with contrast. There was no hydrocephalus and no evidence of a venous sinus thrombosis. The pathergy test was negative.

Diagnosis   Behçet's syndrome

Commentary by Professor David H Miller and Dr Nicholas A Losseff

This man presents with a subacute history of meningism associated with an evolving brainstem syndrome characterised by asymmetric pupils, an internuclear ophthalmoplegia, respiratory depression and eventually a spastic quadraparesis. Of extreme diagnostic importance is his ethnic origin, history of uveitis, family history and the presence of pharyngeal ulceration. If these other features were coincident then a broad differential diagnosis would exist and it would be necessary to consider infections that can attack the brainstem (*Listeria*, TB, herpes simplex, Lyme disease and syphilis) as well as inflammatory causes such as acute disseminated encephalomyelitis, sarcoidosis and Behçet's syndrome. Several diseases can produce uveitis and meningeal disease in addition to sarcoid and Behçet's disease and these include Vogt–Koyanagi–Harada syndrome, Whipple's disease and acute multifocal

146

placoid pigment epitheliopathy. However, in this patient the clinical picture is most suggestive of Behçet's disease and this is supported particularly by the imaging abnormalities, especially the extension of the signal abnormalities into the internal capsules. Behçet's disease is diagnosed on clinical criteria (there being no diagnostic laboratory test) of recurrent oral ulceration (oro-pharyngeal ulceration is far more specific) plus two of the following: recurrent genital ulceration, ocular lesions (venous occlusive disease is addition to uveitis is most suggestive), skin lesions and a positive pathergy test.

In Caucasians the pathergy test is usually unhelpful. CNS involvement occurs in 10–20% of cases with a predilection for the brainstem. Other important CNS manifestations include venous sinus thrombosis, aseptic meningitis, often with an excess of polymorphs, and diencephalic lesions presenting with sudden coma. Rarely a myelopathy, optic neuropathy or behavioural disturbance may be the presenting feature. MRI can reveal striking abnormalities in the pons, midbrain, thalamus and internal capsule, with gadolinium enhancement and swelling in the acute stages. Pathologically, areas of perivascular inflammation and necrosis are seen. Intrathecal synthesis of oligoclonal bands is distinctly unusual. Treatment of acute attacks is with steroids. In the long term, azathioprine may be helpful. Thalidomide produces dramatic resolution of the oropharyngeal ulceration.

Reference

O'Duffy JD, Goldstein NP. Neurologic involvement in seven patients with Behçet's disease. *Am J Med* 1976;**61**:170–8.

Case 46

History	A 22-year-old woman presented with a 1-year history of progressive visual failure. She initially noticed poor vision affecting the left eye followed several months later by more rapidly involving visual loss affecting the right eye. She had also noticed non-specific headaches. She had been born in the UK but had spent the previous 15 years in Nigeria where she had been treated with chloroquine for presumed malaria on several occasions. She had not been prescribed other medications and did not drink alcohol to excess. For 6 months she had also been feeling rather lethargic. There was also a 6-month history of secondary amennorhoea.

Examination

There was anosmia affecting the left nostril. Other abnormalities were confined to the visual system. Visual acuities were reduced bilaterally to perception of light in the inferior nasal fields only. Both pupils were rather dilated (6 mm) and reacted poorly to the direct and consensual light reflex. Fundoscopy revealed bilateral optic atrophy with attenuation of the surrounding vessels.

Investigations

Routine haematology and biochemistry were normal. Thyroid function tests were normal. Oestradiol levels were 85 pmol/l (normal range 100–1400 pmol), and prolactin was 1056 mu/l (normal range <525 mu/l). FSH and LH levels were low. Random cortisol level was normal. CT of the brain and pituitary revealed a large multicystic suprasellar mass with multiple foci of calcification. The mass extended to involve the interpeduncular fossa with mass effect manifested on both frontal lobes and the third ventricle. The lateral ventricles were dilated.

Diagnosis   Craniopharyngioma

Commentary by Dr Gordon T Plant

Craniopharyngioma commonly presents with severe visual loss in children and young adults. Secondary amenorrhoea is common and I have seen patients who have been investigated for this for some years before the onset of visual failure leads to the diagnosis. The pattern of visual loss in craniopharyngioma is variable. There is often a combination of signs indicating involvement of the optic tract, the chiasm and the optic nerve or nerves. A wide range of visual presentations can also occur with pituitary adenomas but straightforward bitemporal hemianopia is much more common than in the case of

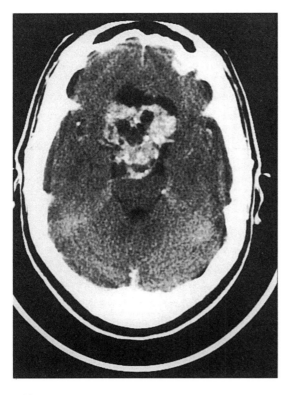

Figure 27
Craniopharyngioma. CT scan showing large multifocal cystic lesion with calcification.

craniopharyngioma. Suprasellar meningioma would be the major third differential diagnosis in this patient. The optic atrophy seems to have been profound and the prognosis for visual recovery must be poor. I am sure that the attenuation of the retinal vessels is entirely secondary to the optic atrophy. Calcification on imaging is an important clue to the ultimate histological diagnosis, this finding seems much less common in older patients (Figure 27). The imaging findings are quite variable in terms of signal characteristics and pattern of enhancement. This patient would soon have experienced problems from a common complication – namely, hydrocephalus.

Reference

Horvath E, Scheithauer BW, Kovacs K, Lloyd RV. Regional neuropathology: hypothalamus and pituitary. In: Graham DI, Lantos PL, Eds. *Greenfield's Neuropathology*, 6th Edn. London: Arnold; 1997:1007–94.

CASE 47

History   A 56-year-old woman had been born in Jamaica and had emigrated to the UK in her teenage years. At the age of 43 years she developed increasing back pain and difficulty walking. Five years later she noticed an insidious onset of urinary urgency and frequency. Her gait continued to deteriorate and she also developed proximal weakness affecting her arms. There was no family history of neurological disorders.

Examination

Abnormalities were confined to the peripheral nervous system. In the upper limbs there was mild wasting and proximal weakness with preserved reflexes and normal tone. Lower limb examination was characterised by a pyramidal pattern of weakness, pathologically brisk reflexes and bilaterally extensor plantars. There was no muscle tenderness or sensory abnormalities.

Investigations

Routine haematology and biochemistry were normal. Thyroid function tests were normal. The creatine kinase level was 336 IU/l (normal range <180 IU/l). Syphilis serology was negative. CSF analysis showed a protein level of 0.61 g/l, 2 lymphocytes, normal glucose level and positive oligoclonal bands (matched with serum). HTLV1 antibodies were positive in serum and CSF. MRI investigation of the cord was normal. Somatosensory and visual evoked potentials were normal. Nerve conduction studies were normal but the EMG was floridly myopathic with frequent fibrillations, positive sharp waves and small spiky polyphasic units of low amplitude and short duration. A muscle biopsy from the right vastus showed denervation changes only.

> **Diagnosis**   HTLV1 associated myelopathy and myopathy

Commentary by Dr Peter Rudge

The above history is typical of that for HTLV1-positive tropical spastic paraparesis with back pain, difficulty walking and urinary disturbance, progressing over 4–5 years. Characteristically, these patients have little or no sensory disturbance. Usually, UK patients have emigrated from the West Indies in their teens or early twenties and develop symptoms after the age of 40 years. The majority are female. The CSF is usually characterised by marginally elevated protein levels and cell counts with positive oligoclonal bands. These are frequently matched with serum and a proportion of the bands recognise antigens from HTLV1. The titres of HTLV1 antibodies in the serum are very high. A substantial number of patients who left the West Indies before the mid-1970s have positive syphilis serology in the serum but it is invariably negative in the CSF. MRI of the cord usually returns a normal signal although there may be associated atrophy. Approximately half of the patients have normal evoked potentials. The interesting feature about this particular case was the proximal weakness of the upper limbs with mild elevation of creatine kinase and EMG evidence of a florid myopathy. However, the biopsy taken from the lower limbs showed no evidence of a myopathy, but merely denervation. In the literature a myositis is well described and is of interstitial type. However, the EMG is not reliable in distinguishing denervation from polymyositis. The absence of a family history is fairly typical of the cases in the United Kingdom although some 10–15% of patients do indeed have other family members who are affected. A substantial number of patients of this type have been seen at the National Hospital over the years and the disease was inappropriately termed 'Jamaican neuropathy'. The pathological brunt of this illness is borne by the dorsal spinal cord, as was first demonstrated by McMenemy in the mid-1960s.

Reference

Cruckshank JK, Rudge P, Dalgleish AG, *et al*. Tropical spastic paraparesis in human T cell lymphotropic virus type 1 in the United Kingdom. *Brain* 1989;**112**:1057–90.

CASE 48

History	A 65-year-old right-handed Ghanaian woman had emigrated to the UK 30 years previously. She had travelled back to Ghana on numerous occasions. Her neurological problems began 5 years previously when her relatives noticed that she had developed a stammer and her speech had become rather non-fluent. Over the next 5 years she experienced a progressive decline in her language skills and would frequently admix Gha and English words in the same sentence. Her reading became affected and her speech entirely nonsensical. Her comprehension skills were relatively preserved and she seemed to have insight into her problems. She had become quite irritable but her family felt that her personality was reasonably unaltered. She had been hypertensive for 10 years but there was no other significant past medical or family history.

Examination

The patient was smartly dressed. Her speech was virtually incomprehensible with frequent neologisms. She was able to obey one-step commands but unable to repeat words or phrases. Her reading skills were markedly impaired but she was able to write, although she made frequent graphemic and syntactical errors. She exhibited a relative preservation of visuoperceptual and visuospatial skills. She had palmomental and pout reflexes but the rest of the neurological examination was normal.

Investigations

Routine haematology and biochemistry were normal. The ESR was 25 mm/hour. Syphilis serology was negative. The autoimmune profile, including ANCA and Ro/La were negative. CSF investigation was normal. An MRI scan of the brain revealed generalised atrophy with the most severe changes in the left temporal lobe. High signal lesions were seen in the cortical white matter and basal ganglia. An EEG was relatively normal but slow waves were seen over the left temporal lobe.

Diagnosis Primary progressive aphasia

Commentary by Dr Nicholas C Fox

Mesulam first described primary progressive aphasia (PPA) in six patients in 1982 and emphasised that this was a clinical syndrome rather than a disease entity. The proposed criteria for PPA include a progressive aphasia, relative sparing of non-verbal cognitive abilities for at least the first 2 years of the illness and preservation of activities of daily living. The aphasia is non-fluent in at least 50% of such cases but it has been argued that the term PPA should be applied only to patients with *non-fluent* aphasia. Subtle word finding difficulties may be the initial symptom and as insight is often preserved the patient may be the first to notice a problem. Neuropsychological deficits may initially be confined to errors on confrontational naming. Comprehension is relatively preserved. The language deficits progress gradually until the patient is mute. Global cognitive deficits develop at a variable stage in this decline. Mesulam estimated that the aphasia remains isolated for an average of 5 years. However, other deficits may be detected by detailed neuropsychological assessment. Reading, writing and calculation are impaired early and orofacial apraxia is common. Neurological examination is otherwise initially normal. The EEG shows left temporal slowing later on. Imaging is quite characteristic with focal atrophy of the left anterior temporal and inferior frontal lobes and hypometabolism in a similar distribution. The non-dominant hemisphere is usually relatively spared but with time atrophy becomes generalised, although it remains asymmetrical. The underlying pathophysiology is heterogeneous with Pick's disease, corticobasal degeneration, and Alzheimer's disease all having been reported; however, most common of all are non-specific changes and Pick's disease. Alzheimer's pathology is relatively rare in PPA, particularly in cases where the aphasia is non-fluent. The prognosis is variable but activities of daily living may be maintained for many years. No specific treatments are available at present.

Reference

Mesulam MM, Weintraub S. The spectrum of primary progressive aphasia. In: Rossor MN, Ed. *Unusual Dementias*. London: Baillière Tindall; 1992:583–609.

CASE 49

History	A 23-year-old man had been well until 2 months prior to admission. At that stage he developed a sore throat and other coryzal symptoms. Three weeks later, whilst seated, he had a sudden onset of nausea, vomiting and rotational vertigo lasting for 2 hours. He was taken to the local casualty department, prescribed antibiotics with an antiemetic and sent home. Since then his balance had become progressively worse and the vertiginous attacks had continued. He also complained of diplopia with no directional preponderance. He was admitted to hospital and over the next week developed a left facial weakness with associated numbness. He had been previously well.

Examination

General examination was normal and he was apyrexial. He had marked truncal and gait ataxia. Visual acuity and fundal examination were normal. There was evidence of an internuclear ophthalmoplegia. In addition, he had upbeat nystagmus that was maximal on upgaze and reduced optokinetic nystagmus to the right. Corneal sensation was reduced on the left. There was a left lower motor neurone facial palsy. There was no evidence of bulbar involvement. In the peripheral nervous system tone, power and reflexes were normal. Both plantar responses were flexor. There was minimal impairment of coordination affecting the left upper limb but no other cerebellar signs.

Investigations

Routine haematology and biochemistry were normal. CSF analysis was normal with negative oligoclonal bands. MRI of the brain revealed evidence of a high signal mass crossing the midline in the region of the corpus callosum (Figure

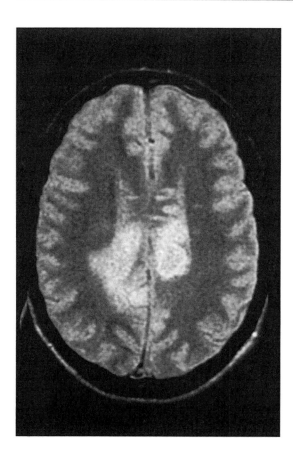

Figure 28 T2 weighted MRI scan showing a high signal lesion crossing the midline.

28). In addition, there were high signal lesions in the left pons and left middle cerebellar peduncle. All the lesions enhanced with contrast. The larger lesion was stereotactically biopsied. Histological features showed a highly cellular tumour consisting of small pleomorphic cells arranged in places to form rosettes. Mitoses were frequent. Staining with synaptophysin antibodies confirmed the neoplasm to be a primitive neuroectodermal tumour (PNET).

Diagnosis   Primitive neuroectodermal tumour

Commentary by Professor Francesco Scaravilli

Primitive neuroectodermal tumours (PNET) are a group of neoplasms consisting of undifferentiated cells with a potential for differentiation into neuronal, glial, muscle and melanotic cells. They occur in the cerebellum as medulloblastomas, although they can also be encountered in the cerebral hemispheres. The view that this term should be extended to all primitive undifferentiated tumours of the central nervous system (CNS) has been opposed by the fact that these entities have already been defined by their site, morphological features and biological behaviour. Medulloblastomas are the commonest and best known variety of PNET; they are malignant, invasive, embryonal tumours of the cerebellum which have a propensity to spread via the CSF. They are second in frequency to pilocytic astrocytomas in children, in whom they account for 20% of CNS neoplasms (2–4% of all brain tumours). The peak incidence is at 3–8 years but 20–25% occur after the age of 20 years. Males are preferentially affected (male:female ratio = 1.6:1). Cases have been reported in identical twins as well as in association with other brain tumours and extraneural malignancies. The commonest location is in the lower portion of the cerebellar vermis but they can also originate from the cerebellar hemispheres, particularly in adults. Embryonal CNS tumours, morphologically indistinguishable from medulloblastomas but located outside the cerebellum, are also included amongst PNET. They are much rarer than medulloblastomas, occurring mostly in children and may be found supratentorially or, in rare instances, in the spinal cord. Histologically they present as highly cellular neoplasms with round or irregularly oval nuclei, scanty cytoplasm and a fibrillary matrix. A high mitotic rate is customary and necrosis or calcification is frequently seen. Supratentorial PNET are thought to originate from the subependymal matrix zones of the lateral ventricles. Neuronal differentiation is indicated by the presence of neuroblastic rosettes. The prognosis of these tumours is usually poor.

Reference

Lantos PL, Vandenberg SR, Kleihues P. Tumours of the nervous system. In: Graham DI, Lantos PL, Eds. *Greenfield's Neuropathology* 6th edn. London: Edward Arnold; 1997:698–710.

CASE 50 (from the archives—1877)

History	'A 42-year-old metalworker was married with one child. His other four children had all died in infancy. He had rheumatic fever and head colic in childhood but had otherwise been well. One year previously he developed a coarse tremor affecting all four limbs. His wife said he looked pale and yellowish and that he frequently complained of paroxysmal colicky abdominal pain lasting several hours. Six weeks prior to admission his wife noticed that he gradually became extremely tremulous and clumsy. He developed word finding difficulties and was unable to recall recent events. This caused him to have some difficulties at work'.

Examination

'He looked older than his years and had arcus senilis. He was pale and thin and a blue line was noted around his gums. His dentition was in an appalling state and his teeth were chipped and decayed. He appeared rather defective and was unable to carry out the simplest commands. He seemed to have some loss of emotional control and was prone to weeping and wailing. His short-term memory was extremely poor and he was unable to give his age. On making him stand upright with his feet together and eyes closed, he swayed very considerably and would have fallen if allowed to do so. Similar signs were noted whilst he was seated. Examination of the cranial nerves revealed an intact first nerve. He was able to read the 8 Snellen with each eye but assessment was difficult as he was an ignorant man and scarcely able to read correctly under the best of circumstances. His third, fourth and sixth cranial nerves were intact with no nystagmus. The fifth cranial nerve was also normal. His seventh nerves seemed strong but when he spoke his facial muscles would quiver markedly. His hearing was excellent and no palatal abnormalities could be detected. His tongue was exceedingly tremulous and his speech was thick and indistinct. He failed to finish his words and often said words different to the ones he intended. He was able to enunciate single words even of moderate complexity (such as comfortable) but on attempted repetition, even after a short time, the word would have no semblance of the original sound. Examination of the spinal nerves was highly informative. He seemed to have very defective power of recovery of the muscles – these muscles remained contracted after he was told to relax. The power in his right arm was rather good but there was an extremely coarse tremor which developed when the arm was extended, being minimal at rest. If his arm was raised and the fingers extended, the tremor became even more marked. Findings in the left arm were similar. Upper limb sensation was normal. Examination of the lower extremities revealed that he was able to walk fairly well and indeed walked up to the hospital from his house (a distance of over 1 mile). He had no trembling of the legs whilst walking. However, after exertion he seemed scarcely able to raise his legs off the chair and developed a coarse tremor. Sensation was normal and he had no sphincter disturbance. Since admission there has been a remarkable improvement though not in his reasoning or memory.'

Diagnosis	Possible general paresis of the insane, possible lead encephalopathy

INDEX

163

164

T - #1065 - 101024 - C0 - 229/152/8 [10] - CB - 9781853176777 - Gloss Lamination